Vital Involvement
in Old Age

Vital Involvement in Old Age

Erik H. Erikson

Joan M. Erikson

Helen Q. Kivnick

W·W·NORTON & COMPANY
New York   London

Published simultaneously in Canada by Penguin Books Canada Ltd.,
2801 John Street, Markham, Ontario L3R 1B4.
Printed in the United States of America.

The text of this book is composed in Times Roman, with
display type set in Tiffany Demi Caps. Composition and
manufacturing by The Haddon Craftsmen, Inc.
Book design by Jacques Chazaud.

First Edition

Library of Congress Cataloging-in-Publication Data
Erikson, Erik H. (Erik Homburger), 1902–
Vital involvement in old age.
Includes index.
1. Aged—Psychology. 2. Life cycle, Human—Longitudi-
nal studies. 3. Aged—United States—Psychology.
I. Erikson, Joan M. (Joan Mowat) II. Kivnick, Helen Q.
III. Title.
HQ1061.E75   1986   305.2'6   86–16380

ISBN 0-393-02359-1

W. W. Norton & Company, Inc., 500 Fifth Avenue, New York, N. Y. 10110
W. W. Norton & Company Ltd., 37 Great Russell Street, London WC1B 3NU

1 2 3 4 5 6 7 8 9 0

Contents

Preface

In our first chapter, we indicate that this book consists of the three authors' "joint reflections" on old age. Here we should perhaps explain what we mean by "joint reflections" and who we three are who are presuming to engage in such reflecting.

Over the last few years, we have had the opportunity (described in detail in Chapter I) of interviewing twenty-nine octogenarians on whom—and especially on whose children —life-historical data had been collected over a period of half a century, by the "Guidance Study" of the Institute of Human Development, of the University of California at Berkeley. Since 1928, the Guidance Study has followed the lives of a large number of children born in Berkeley in 1928 and in the first half of 1929, as these children and their parents have aged through more than five decades. In the nineteen forties, in fact, one of us (EHE) conducted play observations with the "Guidance Study children," then in their early teens, and summarized fifty of their life histories.

That was in the era when Jean Walker Macfarlane provided the leadership and the inspiration for the study and when the octogenarians who are our informants today were the young to middle-aged parents of adolescent children.

We three authors share (if on the basis of different professional experiences and degrees of longevity) a dynamic theory of the ages and stages of human life, from infancy to old age. In Chapter I (Section 4), we spread out before the reader our shared meeting ground, namely, an epigenetic theory of the stages of human life as completed in old age.

This theory has permitted us to integrate our recent interviews with material gathered since 1928, in order to reflect on the "vital involvements" of our aged informants. In Chapter II, we undertake to discuss the experiences and interests of these people, in old age and in earlier life, in an attempt to understand most fully the psychosocial process of "vital involvement" in later life.

We offer the reader, in Chapter III, an exemplary account of one almost completed life history—that of Dr. Borg, the protagonist in Bergman's film *Wild Strawberries.* We have chosen to discuss the life history of a character from this great work of art, rather than that of one of our informants, for two reasons. First, our informants are so few, have participated in the Guidance Study for so long, and are so familiar with the broad outlines of one another's experiences that an intimate description of any one life would unfairly expose that individual to his or her peers. Second, the film we have chosen lends itself particularly well to the consideration of a life history as an integrated whole. Scene for scene, this film describes how an old Swedish doctor, on the long drive to the cathedral of Lund in order to receive a dramatically crowning doctorate, comes to revisit important places of his past and to dream of decisive experiences in his life.

These scenes of a life history "invented" by an insightful genius portray the "logic" and richness of a whole life— including its old age.

After this comprehensive life history, from another decade in a different land, we conclude (in Chapter IV) by discussing some of the more salient issues of old age in our own time and our own country. In this final chapter, we consider major trends in the "fate" of America's elders today, and we draw on our understanding of the life cycle to suggest ways in which this fate might be improved.

About ourselves: Erik H. Erikson is a psychoanalyst and a professor emeritus of human development at Harvard University. He is in his ninth decade. Joan M. Erikson is an artist and a craftswoman who, in such clinical settings as the Austen Riggs Center and the Mount Zion Hospital in San Francisco, has developed a method of using art experience to mobilize dormant strengths in the service of recovery and growth. She, too, is in her ninth decade. Helen Q. Kivnick is a clinical and research psychologist. Her clinical work and her research on grandparenthood, on aging, and on the psychosocial value of participatory arts activities that cut across cultural lines reflect a commitment to the understanding and enhancing of psychosocial health throughout the life cycle. She is nearly fifty years younger than her two colleagues.

We thus are coworkers and coauthors of different ages and differing professional careers; and the reader will probably want to know how we three wrote this one book together. Each chapter, though first intensively discussed by all three, was chosen and written by one of us and then studied and edited by the other two. Finally, the whole book was submitted to our publisher's perceptive editorship, in the person of Linda Healey.

Although the background of the data reported here

reaches far into the past of Berkeley, California, our study depended on the trust and support of leading members of two very contemporary academic and administrative staffs—one in California and one in Pennsylvania. The present director of the Institute of Human Development, at Berkeley, is Prof. Guy E. Swanson; he welcomed and encouraged our research, and his staff were most helpful with our ongoing orientation in this task. Dorothy Eichhorn and Marjorie Honzik, both of whom well understand the nature of our assignment, guided our search. Also of special help were Carol Huffine and Mark Welge. Arden Parish helped us immeasurably with the detailed demands of recording the data from our interviews.

Other forms of support came from the East. Financial support was provided by the National Institute of Mental Health (represented by Gene Cohen and Barry Lebowitz) and by the National Institute of Handicapped Research, by way of the Rehabilitation Research and Training Center of Aging at the University of Pennsylvania, directed by Stanley J. Brody. His and his staff's emphasis on the need for *rehabilitation* in the lives of many old people was particularly useful. His fiscal coordinator, Dolores Foster-Kennedy, ably handled our administrative problems.

Finally, our acknowledgments must extend into our homes. The Eriksons have had to learn further to let home life and research be involved with one another as vitally as could be. For Helen Kivnick, home-based support has come unfailingly from Gary Gardner. He has provided encouragement, humor, and perspective—and we three thank him wholly and heartily.

Vital Involvement
in Old Age

I

Ages
and Stages

I. AN INTRODUCTION

This book consists of joint reflections on old age as the
concluding stage of the life cycle, with continual emphasis on
the vital involvements necessary at each stage, from the first
to the last. Such a life-historical perspective, however, must
always be seen in the context of the stage of history that, at
a given time, dictates the conditions under which an individual gets a chance for age-specific participation in pursuits
essential not only for his and her own development but also
for that of the relatives (and the neighbors) in the same
generational cycle.

Here one could examine the various ways in which old age
has been dealt with throughout the world's history, in different periods and civilizations of the past and the present. But
such historical examination would probably teach us little
about what we want to know most, for history has been
interested primarily in the elite old people—those true "el-

ders" who for one reason or another were revered and ritually buried so as to enter whatever afterlife was, more or less mystically, prescribed. About the great number of less-known old, we could probably only generalize. However, where long-lived elders held the monetary power, the land, and the rank, they were treated accordingly. Today we are faced with an unprecedented growth in the number of so-called elderlies in a technological world in which their over-all role remains quite unclear. There is apparently little historical continuity preserved by their voices and their presence. The fabric of society, the center, "does not hold" the aged.

A good look at the conditions of old age in our stage of history makes it obvious that we are all facing the prospect of a steadily increasing longevity in an unpredictable technological future—a future in which, in fact, it must first be proven that mankind as a whole can survive its own reckless inventiveness. From here on, old age must be *planned,* which means that mature (and, one hopes, well-informed) middle-aged adults must become and remain aware of the long life stages that lie ahead. The future of these long-lived generations will depend on the vital involvement made possible throughout life, if old people are somehow to crown the whole sequence of experience in the preceding life stages. In other words, a life-historical continuity must be guaranteed to the whole human life cycle, so that middle life can promise a vivid generational interplay and old age can offer what we will describe as an existential integrity—the only immortality that can be promised.

Now, to make clear our own involvements, we, the writers of this book, want to state that we have chosen to study, to interview, and to discuss together a number of individuals who are as old as or older than the oldest of us and who have submitted themselves, as they submitted their children, to the "longitudinal" study that we will describe and discuss below. But first we should note how we became involved in this study under different conditions. We belong to a relatively recent school of investigation, namely, that of overall human development. And while two of us share the octogenarian age of our informants, one of us is in the middle of a relatively young adulthood.

As for the historical conditions under which we are working, we should note that since the middle of this century much general interest has been awakened first in child development and then in all ages and stages of life, and this beyond the special clinical interest of "case histories" or of the biographies of individuals of special historical interest. Our subjects are indeed "ordinary" members of a well-known community, namely, Berkeley, California, selected for study merely because their children belonged to a statistical sample born in a certain year. Such a selection of "ordinary" lives, furthermore, could have happened only in our century, in the middle of which the White House Conference on Children was convened, in search of "a healthy personality for *every* child." Indeed, our century has since been named the Century of the Child, for in its early decades an international interest in childhood and in "mental health" was awakened that was to match the interest in the classifiable misadaptations that Freud recognized as being of universal and fateful importance. The special interest in childhood was variously personified in great teachers and scientists like Dewey, Gesell, and Mead in this country and Montessori and Piaget abroad, to whom foundation grants became available thanks to insightful agents like Lawrence K. Frank.

Two of the authors of this book (EHE and JME) contributed to the midcentury conference on children a (then rare) theory of the ("psychosocial") stages of life—a theory that also dominates our present effort and that will be outlined in section 4 of this chapter. Subsequent decades of this century have ushered in an equally general and concentrated interest in other stages of human life: adolescence (and its search for identity) in the 1960s, adulthood in the 1970s, and now old age.

2. The Origins of Our Project

In this matrix of social concern and scientific interest, the Laura Spelman Rockefeller Foundation was approached, and it agreed to fund a longitudinal study of human development at the University of California at Berkeley. This study marked a confluence of several streams of interest. Richard Bolt of Berkeley's Department of Hygiene had established that in the city of Berkeley the rate of infant mortality was exceptionally low, a statistic at once stimulating and surprising. The Thom Clinics and the Department of Pediatrics at the University of California had for some time been trying to identify the early roots of the behavior problems they were observing in their clients. Highly trained and keenly motivated professional workers were available to examine the issues involved. In every regard, the time appeared ripe.

With Herbert R. Stolz, M.D., as director and Harold Ellis-Jones, Ph.D., as director of research, the Institute of Child Welfare was founded in 1927. In that year, it opened one of the first nursery schools in California and completed plans for the "Berkeley Survey," a study of infant health and development that involved every third child born in Berkeley over an eighteen-month period.

In the years immediately following, three major longitudinal studies were in fact established in pursuit of these efforts: the Berkeley Growth Study, the Guidance Study, and the Oakland Growth Study.

Our work, as reported in this book, is based only on the records of the Guidance Study and on our own current interviews with the parents of children who were the subjects of this study.

> The 248 original participants were drawn from a socioeconomic survey of every third birth in Berkeley between January 1, 1928, and June 30, 1929. . . . Despite this selection procedure, the Guidance Study sample differed from the general United States population (as judged by census data) in ways expectable in a university community. Hospital deliveries exceeded the national average, and the infant mortality rate was lower. Although their incomes were below average, the Guidance Study parents were above average in education status and more likely to own their own homes and to have labor-saving appliances.*

The study maintained a comprehensive longitudinal program through the age of eighteen with a remarkable continuity of participation on the part of their original subjects.

Beginning at the age of six months, the Guidance Study babies were visited at their homes by nurses, who reported on their general health. At twenty-one months, the children and their mothers began to make half-yearly visits to the institute. Their health, eating and sleeping habits, and elimination were noted, and their behavior problems were discussed with the mother. The records of these sessions supply intimate data on the family life of our subjects and on their methods of bringing up their children. The regular visits also afforded the interviewers from the Guidance Study the op-

---

*Dorothy H. Eichorn et al., eds., *Present and Past in Middle Life* (New York: Academic Press, 1981), 34.

portunity to help the mother understand her child's needs and to suggest ways of solving the manifold problems of nurturing and child rearing. These visits with the children, focusing on their development, continued for sixteen years and included physical checkups and a variety of tests and measurements. The physical checkups went on for another two years, until the children were eighteen.

When the children were seventeen, in 1945–46, the parents were interviewed alone; the focus then was the parents' own personal lives and problems.

Further funding financed a five-year follow-up. Prof. Jean W. Macfarlane assumed the direction of this study in 1928. In 1938, she published a monograph for the Society for Research in Child Development* describing the nature and scope of the study and listing the following three objectives:†

> *First,* we are contributing further information on the frequency and persistency of problem behavior at different age levels in a representative group of children. . . .
>
> *Second,* we are seeking to investigate relationships between the child's typical behavior whether in the realm of personality make-up or achievement, and his endowments *and* environment, both physical and psychological. . . .
>
> *Third,* we hope to secure information with which we may evaluate certain current assumptions as to the relation between early emotional patterns and subsequent maladjustment. . . .

In 1960 the institute offered an outline, summarized below, describing the extent of the material and the vast quantity of data concerning the family relations that the study recorded

---

*Macfarlane, *Studies in Child Guidance,* vol. 1, *Methodology of Data Collection and Organization,* Monographs of the Society for Research in Child Development, vol. 3, no. 6 (Washington, D.C.: Society for Research in Child Development National Research Council, 1938).

†The fourth objective, dealing with methodology, is too detailed to be included here.

and that are now available to some researchers in this field:

1. Historical and factual data have been brought up to date since the subjects were aged eighteen (for approximately 150 subjects); these regard education, job record, marriage, children, and other major events of the life career.

2. Four intensive interviews are recorded; they focus, respectively, on the periods of high and low morale, relationships with their parents, relationships with their children, and a comparison of their own families with those of their spouses.

3. A longitudinal health record.

4. A test program, including intelligence tests, projective tests, and a test to appraise perceptions of "important others."

"Studies now under way deal with such topics as the predictive significance of early measures, factors associated with change or maintenance of status, three-generation comparisons, assortative mating patterns, and vocational choice and satisfaction. The followup has permitted the

> gathering of a unique body of biosocial and behavior data on adults for whom extensive documentary records were available from infancy. Since it permits detailed analysis of factors in the growing years as they relate to maturity, immaturity, or personality disturbance in adult life, it should provide an appreciable addition to theory and knowledge concerning personality development.*

In the years since 1960, additional funding has increased this wealth of data by permitting follow-up interviews with both the subjects and their parents at various intervals. The

---

*Institute of Human Development archives.

widened scope of research of these studies was acknowledged in 1958 by the Regents of the University of California when they changed the name of the Institute of Child Welfare, the home of these longitudinal studies, to that of the Institute of Human Development.

We three investigators became research associates of the institute in 1981 when we received funding from the National Institute of Mental Health under the auspices of the Rehabilitation Research and Training Center on Aging at the University of Pennsylvania to conduct a study of the parents of the Guidance Study children.

The material most pertinent to our study of the parents was embedded in a mass of information about the children and was not immediately related to our project. However, the initial interview with one or both parents, conducted in 1928 as part of the original Berkeley Survey, had gathered information about their ancestry, occupations, income, housing, and health. There was also information concerning the age and sex and the health and behavior problems or idiosyncrasies of the siblings in the family. This early body of data was of great interest to us, because it provided scanty but important generational information regarding the ethnic and social roots of our subjects.

In 1968, the parents of the now forty-nine-year-old children were again interviewed in the same manner. By 1981, the children were all over fifty, and the remaining parents ranged from seventy-five to ninety-five years of age. All of these records are in the voluminous files. Additional data were also at our disposal.

In the 1940s, Erik H. Erikson was on the staff of the Guidance Study. At that time, he conducted some "play configuration" interviews with all of the children in their early teens.* He also wrote summaries (now in the institute files) of the first decades of fifty children and their family milieus. These summaries contained an abstract of the parents' personalities and child-rearing styles as revealed throughout the years. As we have pointed out, we later selected for our present study the surviving parents of the fifty children then "summarized," for it is of special interest to see now what, on the basis of the data available in the forties, could be predicted about the life course of the children and, by implication, about the old age of the parents. In 1981, then, we elected to base our study of old age on the twenty-nine extant and locally available parents of this group of fifty children, about whom these summaries had been written.

Macfarlane's monograph *Studies in Child Guidance,* mentioned earlier, summarizes the Guidance Study's basic orientation as dedicated to human nature's "zest, adaptability, and stamina." But only a few, if any, other workers would have dared to use such terms—and to use them both believingly and believably—in what she called "the longitudinal study of a normal group of children." Macfarlane apparently meant to emphasize that she wanted to base such a study, not on a quasi-clinical approach like the then so popular "unraveling" of the antecedents of already established maladjustment, but rather on a balanced approach to what she (also) called "the antecedents of already developing, adjustive and maladjustive patterns," and to fuse the study of such devel-

---

*Eventually, the play configurations common to boys and girls, respectively, proved statistically so convincing that Marjorie Honzik (who at that time was already a widely respected researcher on the Guidance Study staff) decided to publish a summary of these observations. It appeared in the *American Journal of Orthopsychiatry* in 1951 and was listed in Harold Jones's *Studies in Human Development,* University of California Research Bulletin, no. 20. Also, it makes up a brief chapter in the second edition of Erik H. Erikson's book *Childhood and Society* (New York: W. W. Norton, 1963).

opmental matters with a cautious guidance of the families. It must be obvious, then, that in offering "guidance" in the very activity of researching the lives of (at least) two inter- locking generations, a study could gain new insights into the nature of life histories as well as into that of developmental issues.

Interview 1

We approached our subjects by writing a letter introduc- ing ourselves, which was cosigned by the director of the Institute of Human Development. On entering our subjects' life spaces for the first interviews, we were welcomed warmly. Such a welcome after their many years of associa- tion with the study indicated that the relationship of our old subjects with the staff of the institute had been and still was a positive one. We were eager to maintain this positive rela- tionship, since we knew that more such demands would be made on these generous people.

For this first interview, we had planned rather run-of-the- mill questions eliciting factual information about family and personal history. All our inquiries were open-ended; when- ever the information we sought was offered in the ongoing process of the conversation, we never pointedly repeated the question. We had no intention of quantifying our data and could be very free with the interview process. Tape recorders made it unnecessary for us to take verbatim notes, and we worded each question as we saw fit to maintain the flow of conversation. Couples were interviewed singly, although it was not always possible to exclude the uninterviewed partner completely. The sessions lasted approximately two hours, although some of the older people (including the Eriksons) grew weary toward the end. We conducted our first inter-

views without having read any of the copious information
about our subjects so that our interest could be genuinely
that of interviewers who were there to become acquainted.

3. Life and Times

Before discussing how we organized the material accrued in
our interviews, we must briefly describe the geographical
space as well as the time in which our subjects have spent
their lives. Because they were born around the turn of the
century, their experience encompasses the history of the
twentieth century to date. We Eriksons were also children of
the century. Our childhoods knew the wonder of the early
years of the 1900s, when the world was different. And the two
of us lived in Berkeley in the late 1930s and experienced some
of the vestiges of its intimate, precity characteristics. We felt
drawn into this background of our subjects' childhoods and
knew the geographical setting of their early lives, for almost
all of them had spent those years in the Bay Area or in
Berkeley itself. It was not difficult for us to visualize pre–
First World War Oakland and Berkeley—no bridges, very
few cars, and many clanking trolleys—for we had also experienced small-town growing up in the same decades. We,
too, had been close to real needs—simple bodily needs like
food and clothes and the need not to waste materials and
things. In those days, there was space: empty lots where you
played and where wildflowers grew, and safe, half-empty
streets that got very muddy in winter. There was scope for
initiative. You could still sell door-to-door and peddle
bunches of flowers and glasses of lemonade (in the shade). A
nostalgic septuagenarian recollects how beautiful Berkeley
was at that time: "When we were children, you know, we
could play baseball and football in empty lots. That was what

they were for—empty lots—and we could hit the ball as hard as we wanted, and it didn't matter or break anybody's windows." Old Berkeleyans could remember grandparents who lived on what are now town or small-city streets and had manure piles in front of their houses. Cows could graze in backyards; there were chickens and cocks that crowed at dawn. The boys all had jobs delivering papers or performing other services after school. "On a bicycle I would deliver drugs and prescriptions and things of that kind." "I pulled weeds for the city of Berkeley." "I got a dollar a day" (for working in a garden). Girls helped at home with household chores. "We washed our own clothes and ironed them, and we had the dishes to do." There was hope and enterprise, and our old people had as children sensed this and remember their early years as shiny and vital: "They were good times —there was no traffic and few policemen."

The first cataclysmic event in their young lives would have been the First World War. Except for two of our men, it did not seem to be a topic of major reminiscence. The Great War is remembered as a period of some excitement, but the major events took place far away, and even the news of them reached the West Coast slowly.

The Great Depression was a challenging experience of a different order. These were for them the later years of schooling or the early years of marriage and child raising. To achieve and maintain family independence was a major struggle. A number of the young families shared householding with parents who could make space for them. The move into a house of one's own later on was a prideful step toward greater independence and individuation.

Like the quest for housing, the finding and keeping of work was difficult during the Depression. It required both initiative and competence. "I'd get a job, and it would run out and I'd find something else—I can't even remember everything I did." When work was available, it meant long, arduous hours. "We worked eighteen hours a day, sometimes twenty. Our children, when they were small, just kind of grew up. They would fix their own dinners and make their own beds." A number of our subjects felt obliged to drop out of school. "My mother was a widow, and it was pretty hard for her to keep shoes on all of us—so I quit school." They were hard years, remembered in terms like these: "I wouldn't want to go through that again. It was rough."

However, the Second World War changed Berkeley and the lives of our subjects drastically. The shipyards, the oil companies, and the presence of military and naval personnel increased the population immensely. The Bay Bridge connecting Berkeley with San Francisco had just been opened. Jobs were available for men and women, and it was appropriate and patriotic to work. Although the children of the study were too young to serve in World War II, many had siblings who did, and radio and harbor activities kept the area connected and involved with current events. The interviews of 1945 with our subjects, the parents of the Guidance Study children, reflect this excitement and their adaptation to the changes in Berkeley itself.

The presence of a major university in Berkeley, one that had grown impressively in both size and eminence during the years of our subjects' adulthood, had a strong impact on their lives. Only a few of them "made it" to the university them selves, but many of their children were students there, and it was a lively presence in many ways. It is interesting to report, however, that the years of student unrest and excitement that upset the campus in the late sixties, and changed the environs of the university almost unrecognizably, made few headlines with our informants. They personally had few ties to the institution, and their children were for the most part married and had settled into the "maintenance of the world." Our subjects spoke disparagingly of the rebellious behavior of the students and the general unrest and irresponsibility of the young, but the events did not appear to have disturbed them personally in any threatening way.

Throughout all this, we later learned in the Guidance Study records of family problems—of difficulties physical and/or emotional with the children which escalate in critical importance during their high school years. There were marital problems, too, although only one of our subjects was divorced. There were also serious illnesses that inflicted sadness and great strain on old and young alike. Our subjects, then, had survived a gamut of human suffering and were, when we talked with them, somehow integrating this past with an appropriate withdrawal from strenuous activity.

Our subjects spoke clearly and interestingly about their lives, not seeming to hold back. When, however, we later learned about some of the crises they had met, the major challenges they had faced with their children and one another, we marveled at the quiet, rather bland way in which they had presented these experiences to us, if they mentioned them at all. A number of times, a blanket statement quietly covered years of problematic relationships: "There have been no problems with the children." "We have had no marital disagreements." These family confrontations involved such traumatic experiences as the disabling effect of a child's illness and death, the extreme delinquency of an adolescent son or daughter, or marital discord that threatened divorce. We made little effort to draw out our informants on subjects they elected to bypass or treat as insignificant, since it was our goal to understand these people in terms of the conflicts they deemed important at this stage of life and chose to discuss.

Personal Space

This very brief summary of the social and historical contexts of our subjects' development leads us to the consideration of how older people arrange for the space in which they wish to live as couples, as part of a family, or alone. Any habitation that one enters as a visitor or an observer always has its ambience, its tone. It is not readily analyzable but is a perception on the visitor's part, Michael Polanyi has called this a tacit knowledge and appreciation of the values of those who have chosen the space, arranged the furniture, and designed the decor. The space inhabited by the individual is an investiture of preferences and usages. For what kinds of activities is it arranged? Is the interior planned as space in which to receive and to welcome others? Does it on the whole suggest dependence on others, or is the space clearly managed by its occupant? Is it full of memorabilia from the past, or does it perhaps immediately draw attention to the generational involvement of its tenant or tenants by displaying the current photographs of the young of the family?

These outward signs of involvement are always on view and perhaps especially in the homes of older people when the social and personal need to "make a statement" with the milieu is less important than previously.

We feel, therefore, that the arrangement of the spaces in which our people live is in many ways as much an indication of their involvement as any verbal statement they made in the course of our interviews. And so we planned to pay special attention to what the general housing arrangements of our small but rather random sample of Berkeley might be. That they were still in the area was one essential element in our selection.

Nearly one-half of the people in our sample live not only

within the precincts of the city itself but even in the house they have occupied throughout their adult lives. One couple actually lives in the house in which one of them was born! Having spent a few years elsewhere, they returned to this house to care for an aging parent and then remained there.

Five subjects had selected homes for their old age in retirement communities in surrounding areas. These are fairly luxurious developments with extra amenities like swimming pools, club rooms, and ample parking facilities. Five widows live in small apartments, and one shares hers with a sister also widowed. One woman lives in her daughter's house, and one man occupies a small cabin alone. One couple occupies two rooms in a government-subsidized, partial-care facility where personal life-style is somewhat restricted. Another woman lives alone in a retirement apartment building that offers meals and a number of other entertainment and care facilities. As we mentioned earlier, all of our informants live in Berkeley, a milieu in itself, or within a few hours' driving distance. For purposes of this discussion, it is possible to divide them into three categories: the couples (ten individuals), single men (five), and single women (fourteen).

The houses are for the most part neatly maintained, usually with some extra daytime help. We had the feeling that most of the furnishings have been neither replaced nor refurbished. Older people seem to enjoy their old things the way they are. More-recent additions in many cases include the display of family photographs, which are easily at hand when grandchildren are under discussion. Where the men live alone in these houses, fewer pictures are visible; in fact, there is in general less ornamentation, less bric-a-brac. With few exceptions, things are orderly and solid, and few bright colors distract the eye from the view through the windows.

Where the women live alone in these old houses, more "niceties" and articles are on display. For the most part, the colors are clearer and lighter; the arrangement of furniture, more inviting for possible visitors.

Only one of the men offered refreshment of any kind. Almost all of the women made some such gesture of hospitality.

In most of the small apartments, all of which were occupied by women, we were struck by the evident concern of those who had moved into these diminished living areas to keep together old, familiar things. The furniture appeared oversize for the space; many objects, useful perhaps in their own right, seemed, because of the constriction of space, simply to make things look cluttered. This supportive continuity that familiar objects offer us as we age can, of course, be a solace and a pleasure. If they take over today's space too completely, they can also present a problem. However, two of the cluttered rooms we observed showed every sign of ongoing activity so lively that there was nothing stuffy or stifling about them.

Many things quickly became obvious as we were received into these spaces. They breathed a tangible vitality and warmth, or they were maintaining themselves in a faded kind of undemanding way.

Interview 2

The second interviews, in general, were both more difficult to design and more rewarding to conduct than the first. The rapport we had already established made the preliminaries less time consuming, and our information from the longitudinal records and previous interviews allowed us to pose our questions in a way not possible earlier. In an attempt to gather as much information as possible to clarify each of the psychosocial themes, we had prepared our questions to address both old-age and earlier-life experiences related to each theme. This series was quite long, and we did not always try to complete it. Rather, we encouraged our subjects to speak as fully as possible about whatever questions seemed to spark their interest.

The Eriksons found it natural to share "dated" expressions, to joke about their Victorian backgrounds, and to draw out early memories by offering an occasional one of their own. Gestures, laughter, and tone of voice in many cases triggered a feeling of warm empathy. On the other hand, some informants, perhaps out of habit (they had, after all, been interviewed a number of times over the years), gave the initial information or told the same experiences all over again.

As a member of a generation too young to have any firsthand familiarity with the world that our subjects inhabited for the first half of their lives, Helen Kivnick had the advantage of listening to each individual's experiences with a fascination at their difference from anything she knew. She reports, "I could not offer comparable experiences of my own; neither did I pose a standard of comparison or judgment. As I found to be true in my earlier work in open-ended interviews with the elderly, I seemed to elicit in these aged subjects the kinds of warm, concerned, trusting feelings they express for their grandchildren. Where subjects who are my contemporaries may hesitate to express deeply held social, political, or religious convictions unless they know what my views are, these aged subjects did not hesitate at all, often seeming to feel that they were passing on valuable advice in sharing their personal views with me. Where my contemporaries may hesitate to express extreme sadness or pleasure (reluctant to pose explicit comparisons between their lives and mine), or to describe possible outlandish or implausible experiences (reluctant to invoke a judgment of 'crazy'), these elders showed no such hesitation. Uniformly, they responded to my sincere interest in what they had to say—about historical eras and life cycle stages with which I have had no direct contact."

In almost all instances, we each established relationships of real warmth with our informants, so that we were reluctant to say a final good-bye. A few of our elders, on the other hand, we were sure, felt that over the years they had answered enough questions.

In this introduction to the history of the study of which we are a part, we may have raised too high the reader's expectations of what we can deliver. The rare longitudinal data at our disposal and the relative openness of our subjects' welcome may well be perceived as giving us a chance to present rare and intimate data in support of our conclusions regarding the dynamics of their lives and especially of their old age—data more instructive regarding "typical" lives than can be offered in clinical case histories carefully planned and of necessity radically disguised or in biographical life histories of already well-known individuals. However, our letter of introduction to our subjects was accompanied by a signed reiteration of our promise of utmost discretion as the very condition of their participation in the study. We cannot, therefore, offer our readers whole life histories of any of the persons who have been part of this study over the years. However, we do explore specifically our informants' involvements with this last stage of life, and we draw on our knowledge of their earlier histories to elucidate many aspects of their lives today.

In addition, we will take up later in this book a life history that has to us, and to many audiences, for years seemed most illustrative of our approach to the dynamics of life, namely, that of Dr. Isak Borg, as depicted dramatically in Ingmar Bergman's *Wild Strawberries*. Great artists, after all, understand life and know how to make it understood by their work in a way that brings out such deeper meanings of human life as we can approach only theoretically.

So we will now present the theoretical backbone of our overall concept of human life, namely, the "epigenetic" sequence of the main developmental stages, with special emphasis on psychosocial development—the stages of which will appear with special clarity in Bergman's pictorial account of an old man's recovery from a lifelong tendency to disinvolvement.

4. STAGE FOR STAGE: EPIGENESIS

Dynamic Balance of Opposites

The developmental stages to be listed here have, it may seem to some, been listed often enough. This time, though, we want to relate them to major problems in vital involvement—and to relate vital involvement to these stages. We emphasize *vital,* because the mere word *involvement* can have many connotations, good and bad. More often than not, it has some sense of a complex and passive overinvolvement (sometimes even a helpless or hopeless one) from which one cannot free oneself. But nothing could better clarify its "original" meaning than a built-in linguistic alliteration, for in*volve*ment is related to the prenatal containment in our mother's *vulva,* where, modern research suggests, we were not just passively wrapped up but already had to prove our truly "inborn" capacity for involvement, which means our being alive, by stimulating the "environment" as it stimulates us; for as we become vitally involved, we are also challenging the "environment" to involve us in its convincing ways. It is this psychological and social e-volve-ment that is newly extended in each stage of life, at first in close relations to the psychobiological growth that dictates the basic sequence of step-by-step development.

Here we intend to follow through only this one trend, namely, the eight stages of psychosocial development, which produce the strengths necessary for a mutual involvement in an ever-increasing social radius, from infancy through adulthood and into old age. And this is our basic interest in this study: the remaining or new potentials of the last interactions and the vital (if paradoxical) involvement in the necessary disinvolvements of old age.

First, however, we must, for each of the major stages of development, propose two seemingly contrary dispositions, which are here called *syntonic* and *dystonic,* although vital involvement depends on their balance. The first two, in infancy, are a sense of trust and a sense of mistrust: their balance, we claim, helps create the basis for the most essential overall outlook on life, namely, hope, which must be awakened by our primal, our maternal, caretaker(s). To simply list a few further stages, and to give an initial impression of the direction of early development: the second stage is that of early childhood, which must give form to the fruitful opposition of a (syntonic) sense of autonomy and a (dystonic) one of shame and doubt, which together help establish the beginnings of the basic strength of will; the third stage is the play age, which fosters the balance between a sense of initiative and a sense of guilt.

All of the terms used here are admittedly "adult" ones, in

that they really describe what eventually becomes of those earliest dispositions, whereas their original experience can hardly be described in words—a reality that helps make the observation of children so fascinating. Whatever we call them in our adult terms, however, we can see that these early psychosocial trends are related to other developmental facts, such as the psychosexual stages first discovered by Freud, who was thus one of the true originators of the general theory of childhood stages. In infancy, this is the oral (we would add "and sensory") stage of the libido, which provides the necessary instinctual energy for the first psychosocial involvement; early childhood puts the energy first localized in the anal (and we would add "and muscular") libidinization at the disposal of psychosocial involvements. Together, these developments provide for humankind the first basic dispositions necessary for mutual involvement within a widening social radius: hope is, or eventually comes to be, the enduring belief in the benevolence of fate, in spite of the dark urges and rages that also mark the beginning of existence. Hope thus is the ontogenetic basis of faith, being nourished by the maternal faith that pervades the initial patterns of care. *Will,* in turn, comes to be the unbroken determination to exercise free choice as well as self-restraint, in spite of the unavoidable early experience of shame and self-doubt. A maturing will, and the recognition of its limitations, is the basis for the eventual acceptance of law and necessity and is rooted in the judiciousness of parents guided by the spirit of law.

The third stage is the play age, when out of the toying use of the thing world, as well as from fantasy life, there emerges a set of idealized goals and thus the power of eventual purpose. *Purpose* is the courage to envisage and pursue valued goals uninhibited by the defeat of infantile phantasies, by an imposed sense of guilt, and by the fear of punishment.

Derived from the interacting examples of the basic family, it later invests ideals of action.

The next and concluding stage of childhood is the school age. But before offering further definitions of the maturing strengths that guide us to and beyond adulthood, we will do well to chart all the stages in what we have called their epigenetic sequence (see Chart 1). With this design before us, we may proceed beyond early childhood and the play age, to the school age, when the main productive tension is that between syntonic industry—that is, being industrious in order to learn techniques required by the technological system one is to grow into and in order to accomplish more and more advanced tasks—and inferiority. The gradually resulting strength is competence, the free exercise of dexterity and intelligence in the completion of tasks, unimpaired by a forever threatening sense of inferiority. Competence becomes the basis for cooperative participation in technologies and relies, in turn, on the logic of tools and skills. The dominant dystonic disposition of this stage threatens with a pervasive sense of failure.

There follows adolescence, with its basic tensions between the development of a sense of psychosocial identity and its interplay with an unavoidable identity confusion. As this tension gets resolved, a sense of fidelity emerges both toward one's own accruing identity and toward some overall orientation that helps unify one's identity with an existing or emerging ideological world image. This can be formulated thus: *fidelity* is the ability to sustain loyalties freely pledged in spite of the inevitable contradictions of value systems. It is the cornerstone of identity and receives inspiration from confirming ideologies and affirming companionships.

And now for adulthood. The ideological commitment of adolescence, it is to be hoped, will lead to intimate associa-

CHART I: PSYCHOSOCIAL STAGES OF LIFE

	1	2	3	4	5	6	7	8
Old Age								Integrity vs. Despair. WISDOM
Adulthood							Generativity vs. Self-absorption. CARE	
Young Adulthood						Intimacy vs. Isolation. LOVE		
Adolescence					Identity vs. Confusion. FIDELITY			
School Age				Industry vs. Inferiority. COMPETENCE				
Play Age			Initiative vs. Guilt. PURPOSE					
Early Childhood		Autonomy vs. Shame, Doubt. WILL						
Infancy	Basic Trust vs. Basic Mistrust. HOPE							

tions and eventually to patterns of close co-living; for that reason, we would define the dominant tension in young adulthood as that between intimacy and isolation. Intimacy, of course, is more than a variety of intimacies; it is the capacity for eventual commitment to lasting friendships and companionship in general and, in particular, for the genital mutuality suggested in Freud's theory of psychosexuality. Here one other, ever so important (and first adult) strength is love, about which we may say the following: love is mutuality of devotion forever subduing the antagonisms inherent in divided function. It pervades the intimacy of individuals and is thus the basis of ethical concern as elaborated in affiliative patterns.

So now, at last, we come to the adult reality in the world in which generativity within the cross-generational setting of the technologies and cultures must "take care" of what is being procreated, produced, and created. This vital strength of *care* (as we have formulated it) is the widening concern for what has been generated by love, necessity, or accident; it overcomes the ambivalence arising with irreversible obligation. Thus, care attends to the needs of all that has been generated.

And then, indeed, we really come to the last stage, with which we are trying to deal, above all, in our attempts to reflect on and to learn from our present study. Will we be able to use and to confirm what in regard to the last stage we have formulated so far, although our formulations contain such high terms as *integrity* and *wisdom?* Integrity, we suggested, now is and must be the dominant syntonic disposition, in search of balance with an equally pervasive sense of despair. As for the final strength, wisdom, we have formulated it thus: *Wisdom* is detached concern with life itself, in the face of death itself. It maintains and learns to convey the integrity of experience, in spite of the decline of bodily and mental functions.

Development in Time

Any theory concerning the course of life takes a number of overall space-time perspectives for granted and so makes it necessary, and often difficult, for the reader to keep the total image alive while trying to clarify the terms used. Shakespeare, that most sublime of playwrights, had it "all made," in that he could conceptualize "all the world" as a stage—the very circumscribed setting of which he himself was the unchallenged master—while he proceeded to call "ages" what we refer to as stages. We, however, in combining a large number of concepts that have been used to describe this or that stage of life, are using the term *life cycle* for the whole sequence and, it so happens, can make plausible only toward the very end of our presentation why this is, indeed, an intergenerational cycle.

In the meantime, we are continuing to spread out "our" stages in the form of the epigenetic chart that it is now time to present to the reader, or to remind him of. The subtitle of this section, "Epigenesis," expresses our task quite naturally, for *epi* can mean "above" in space as well as "before" in time, and in connection with *genesis* can well represent the space-time nature of all development. Each of the squares that form the diagonal of our chart then names, as we saw, a pair of syntonic *and* dystonic predispositions. Trust is mandatory: but, as we saw, it can exist positively only in juxtaposition with a "sensible" mistrust—also necessary for existence. Only out of a kind of creative balancing of these two tendencies can hope develop. A constant keeping in scale of trust and mistrust remains normative and what we have also called *sympathic* for every stage and for the whole life cycle. On the chart, this aspect of development appears in the vertical that leads to and arises from each square on the diagonal.

Incidentally, such terms as *sensible, creative balancing,* and *keeping in scale* may seem to suggest primarily cognitively conscious and, as it were, intentional processes. However, we refer here to a complex of processes that can be partly conscious and partly unconscious—processes that the individual may have "a sense of" but to which he or she by no means necessarily gives deliberate direction. As the reader may have sensed, all of this has much to do with an individual's central mental tendency to organize experience, which in psychoanalysis has been extensively discussed under the heading of the integrative function of the ego and, in fact, has led to the development of an ego psychology. In each developmental stage, the individual thus experiences a creative tension between the two opposites, a tension that attracts both instinctive and instinctual energy, while the widening radius of interpersonal relations leads, at each stage, to that contact with new sections of the social order, which thus provide, even as they depend on, individual development.

The epigenetic chart also rightly suggests that the individual is never struggling only with the tension that is focal at the time. Rather, at every successive developmental stage, the individual is also increasingly engaged in the anticipation of tensions that have yet to become focal and in reexperiencing those tensions that were inadequately integrated when they were focal; similarly engaged are those whose age-appropriate integration was then, but is no longer, adequate. Consider the early-childhood tension of autonomy versus shame and doubt. Clearly, a healthy two-year-old sense of autonomy must somehow be modified if it is to become a family-tolerated autonomy, a healthy school-age autonomy, a young-adulthood autonomy, and a generative adult and an old-age self-determination. It is this modification to which we refer in postulating a school-age reintegration of, and an appropriate old-age reinvolvement with, this theme. At each successive stage, earlier conflicts must be reresolved in relation to the current level of development.

Thus, the principle of reexperiencing suggests that the old-age struggle appropriately to deal with the tension between integrity and despair depends very largely on an individual's age-appropriate balancing of earlier psychosocial tensions, and also on his or her current resynthesis of all the resilience and toughness of the basic strengths already developed. Yet, the final focal effort to come to terms with integrity and despair is not predetermined or foreclosed by the way life has been lived up to this point. An essential aspect of what is involved in integrating the final two opposites is a renewed and old-age-specific willingness to remember and review earlier experiences.

Maldevelopment

In view of our concern to present the stagewise working patterns of epigenetic development, it is time to take cognizance of what may *not* work in all this balancing. But the immense literature and the many "schools" of psychopathology make it seem best in this context to abstain from specific diagnostic discussions and to indicate merely the "maldevelopments" and malignancies that lessen one's chance to be "vitally involved" in one's life. Our general impression is that if there is a tendency to overdo and to overdevelop the syntonic predisposition in an attempt to let the dystonic wither away, the result may be some maladaptation; and in the case of an overemphasis on the dystonic with a threatening loss of the syntonic, the result may be a turn toward malignancy. As the terms suggest, a maladaptation could eventually be corrected by readaptation, spontaneous or therapeutically induced; a "trend" toward malignancy, by contrast, may lead into a deadlock calling for a more radical correction: clinicians would say that in the first case one would obviously expect a more "neurotic" disturbance and in the second a more "psychotic" one. (The nature of these disbalances is, for each stage, listed in Chart 2.)

If, in the wake of a failure of integration, too much trust results in the first stage, this can, as we have indicated, lead to a maladaptive disorientation, though it is one that retains a chance of being readapted sooner or later. If, however, mistrust remains unbalanced, there can occur a deep trend to withdrawal and thus, sooner or later, a malignant avoidance of involvement, which in many case histories of borderline-psychotic disturbances can indeed be traced back to the first stage of life.

In view of its decisive character, we may well briefly review once more some of the infantile dynamics involved here. The survival of infants depends on their innate trust in their own senses and in the trustworthiness of their caretakers. It is the function of the infant's genetically programmed senses to instigate sensible protest on the part of the whole system when, for example, the food offered is inappropriate in texture, smell, taste, or temperature. Protest, loud or whimpering, is also adaptive if care is less than adequate. An ailing or sense-deprived infant will demand more intimate and personalized attention than a robust one in order to establish adequate trust in his or her caretakers, so that some sensory deprivation may be offset. Where only bare survival is achieved, the infant may resort to a form of more or less malignant withdrawal, which makes life possible but leaves hope weak and unsustaining. Without enough trust in the senses or in the caretakers, there is no source of hope, and the infant cannot survive (as René Spitz has documented). We can therefore assume that all surviving infants have a modicum of trust to build on—trust that may be increased and strengthened with resulting hopefulness to mitigate the ever-present pull of mistrust.

For somewhat older infants who develop an overdependently trusting relationship with overzealous caretakers, such trustful overcompliance may be maladaptive when it is contraindicated by their own sensory perception. This maladaptation could take the form of overrestriction, malnourishing, or adult demands for physical achievement beyond the child's sensed capabilities, such as overstimulation to walk before the muscles are adequately developed.

The senses must appropriately signal mistrust of overstimulation or overcare that endangers the normative cycles of rest and activity and the ingestion of nourishing food. Understimulation of the senses and neglect in caring with little or no mutuality between caretaker and infant may, on the other hand, also set off antipathic tendencies, which can later become malignantly irreversible. In addition, a mistrust of one's own sensory antennae in early life can be the touchstone of future antipathic tendencies and dependencies. Finally, we must note that the full pathological impact of serious antipathic tendencies, in any stage, may become overt only in the next generation.

For the second stage, that of early childhood, we would name as the potential maladaptive trend a (more or less) "shameless" willfulness; and as the result of an intensification of shame and/or doubt a malignant inclination toward severe compulsive self-doubt.

In the third, the play age, an initiative not balanced by a sufficiently empathic capacity for guilt may condone an all too guiltless ruthlessness (and eventually a militant self-extension), while an excessive tendency toward guilt and thus an impairment of purpose may result in a malignant self-inhibition.

Now, to the school age, when a certain integration between an inner readiness to learn and society's readiness to involve the child in schooling must form the basis for competence. In the case of a marked disbalance, industriousness can turn into a "narrow virtuosity" that, for the "whole child," can prove to be a maladaptation, which with some readiness may be readapted by a truly expanded educational experience. For this it is necessary, however, that the habitual inclination toward a sense of inferiority has not led to a potentially malignant state of inertia.

The dangers of some maladaptive and of malignant trends are almost too obvious in adolescence. It is therefore important to state their normative significance. That an adolescent must suffer from role, or identity, confusion and must repudiate some "foreign" values in order to focus his or her beliefs on some chosen ideology—all this is almost too easily criticized, or accepted. At stake in it all is a core of functioning fidelity, which must not disintegrate into a maladaptive fanaticism or a malignant repudiation of otherness.

For young adulthood, we have simply named love as the adaptive strength that should now emerge from all preadult stages—now that the true capacity for selective intimacy replaces all the experimental intimacies of sexuality, friendship, and companionship or, indeed, a painful isolation. The maladaptive danger now is a promiscuous "loving," while the threatening malignancy is a self-isolating and hate-filled exclusivity.

In middle adulthood, love further matures to the care and caring-for that must guide what now, with those one loves, can be procreated, produced, or created—all of which depends on the maturation of generativity. Its dystonic counterpart is stagnation in one or all of these potential involvements. The maladaptation of this stage is an overextension of care to individuals and concerns beyond one's capacity to include; the dominant malignancy now is a generalized rejectivity, which simply does not care to care—for anybody.

As for the extension to old age of this discussion of stagewise maldevelopments and malignancies, the terms we use for a syntonic integrity and a dystonic despair, as well as the suggested dominant strength of wisdom, are so demanding that it seems appropriate to wait until we know more of the vital and not-so-vital involvements of the last phase of life.

Communal Involvement

Even in the relationship of partners of experience as unequal as the newborn and its mother, our formula of "vital" demands that their original involvement in each other be a mutual relationship of a certain reciprocated intensity. Furthermore, if we want to characterize it as a "real" relationship, *real* must mean not only that it is mutually fitting in its "factual" dimension but also that it brings about a special mutualized actuality, that is, an active state keeping awake in both a readiness to develop those patterns of interaction that are ready in each one developmentally—and that means not only in the immediate demands of their respective stages of life but also in an increased readiness for further developments in their future lives. A vitally involved infant is ready not only for the experience of being mothered but also for the development of the conditions basic for an identification with

CHART 2

	Maladaptive Tendency	Adaptive Strength			Malignant Tendency
I.	(Sensory Mal- adjust- ment)	Trust	HOPE	Mistrust	(With- drawal)
II.	(Shameless Will- fulness)	Autonomy	WILL	Shame/ Doubt	(Compul- sion)
III.	(Ruthless- ness)	Initiative	PURPOSE	Guilt	(Inhibition)
IV.	(Narrow Virtuo- sity)	Indus- trious- ness	COM- PETENCE	Inferiority	(Inertia)
V.	(Fanaticism)	Identity Cohesion	FIDELITY	Role Confusion	(Repu- diation)
VI.	(Promis- cuity)	Intimacy	LOVE	Isolation	(Exclu- sivity)
VII.	(Over- extension)	Generativity	CARE	Stagnation	(Rejectivity)
VIII.	(Pre- sumption)	Integrity	WISDOM	Despair	(Disdain)

the mother—and the lifelong capacity to act "maternally."

But all this demands already in the events of infancy a readiness on the part of both participants—that is, participants in each other's lives—a readiness for some cultural variation of experience, which we call *ritualization.* For this term, too, we offer some quotations that in fact put the whole matter of mutual involvement in the necessary context of both evolution and cultural history:*

> We should . . . begin by postulating that behaviour to be called ritualization in man must consist of an agreed-upon interplay between at least two persons who repeat it at meaningful intervals and in recurring contexts; and that this interplay should have adaptive value for both participants. And, I would submit, these conditions are already fully met by the way in which a human mother and her baby greet each other in the morning. . . .
>
> . . . If observed for several days it becomes clear that this daily event is highly ritualized, in that the mother seems to feel obliged, and not a little pleased, to repeat a performance which arouses in the infant predictable responses, encouraging her, in turn, to proceed. Such ritualization, however, is hard to describe. It is at the same time highly *individual* ("typical for this mother" and also tuned to the particular infant) and yet also *stereotyped* along traditional lines [within the given culture]. The whole procedure is superimposed on the periodicity of physical needs close to the requirements of survival; but it is an *emotional* as well as a *practical* necessity for both mother and infant. And, as we will see, this enhanced routine can be properly evaluated only as a small but tough link in the whole formidable sequence of generations. . . .
>
> . . . Daily [as well as cultural] observations (confirmed by the special aura of Madonna-and-Child images) suggest that this

---

*From E. H. Erikson, "Ontogeny of Ritualization in Man," in "A Discussion on Ritualization of Behavior in Animals and Man," organized by Sir Julian Huxley, F.R.S., in *Philosophical Transactions of the Royal Society of London,* ser. B, vol. 251 (1966): 337–49.

mutual assignment of very special meaning is the ontogenetic source of one pervasive element in human ritualization, which is based on a *mutuality of recognition.*

There is much to suggest that man [erect and face-to-face-oriented] is born with the need for such regular and mutual affirmation and certification: we know, at any rate, that its absence can harm an infant radically [for example, in autistic children], by diminishing or extinguishing his search for impressions which will verify his senses [and thus, make sense]. But, once aroused, this need will reassert itself in every stage of life as a hunger for ever new, ever more formalized and more widely shared ritualizations and, eventually, grand rituals which repeat such face-to-face "recognition" of the hoped-for, . . . as in a leader's "charisma" [and a god's "grace"]. I would suggest, therefore, that this first and dimmest affirmation, this sense of a *hallowed presence,* contributes to man's grand *ritual-making* a pervasive element which we will call the "Numinous". This designation betrays my intention to follow the earliest into the last: and, indeed, we vaguely recognize the numinous as an indispensable aspect of periodical *religious observances* [in human history], where the believer, by appropriate gestures, confesses his dependence and his childlike faith and seeks, by appropriate offerings, to secure a sense of being lifted up to the very bosom of the supernatural which in the visible form of an image may graciously respond, with the faint smile of an inclined face. The result is a sense of *separateness transcended,* and yet also of individual *distinctiveness confirmed.*

Let us, finally, list (in an order that can be checked on Chart 1) the new involvements dictated by development at each stage, from the first to the last. And let us begin by listing for each age group a stage of psychosexual development, for our division into childhood stages was, as we said, originally based on Freud's libido theory, which taught us that the strong drive necessary for each new set of basic involvements in childhood and beyond is psychobiologically invigorated by the libidinal instinctuality providing pleasura-

ble experiences as associated with the need for physical satia-
tion. The first stage, orality, clearly demonstrates, in addition
to the maturation of the capacity to suck fluids from such a
preordained source as the maternal person's nipple—or its
artificial substitute—an absorbing erotic pleasure that "naturally" supports the need for intake stimulated and met by
maternal behavior. This mutual involvement leads to the
existentially basic experience of lively trust and some (also
adaptive and unavoidable) mistrust. But, as we now want to
emphasize systematically, all this also calls for specific ritualized forms of parental behavior that are culturally determined. And it also serves, in addition to an immediate adaptation, the establishment of the image of the primal other,
which remains basic for a lifelong sense of hope as being,
stage for stage, attached to the images of vital others and
climaxed by the crowned or otherwise haloed others in the
worldly order—and on up to the ultimate other in a belief
system maintained by faith. Indeed, we will attempt to make
it plausible that man's long and intensive infancy forms the
basis of a forever hoped-for constituent order of man's communal matrix.

Correspondingly, the second stage, early childhood, a
world now experienced also in terms of muscular and anal-
urethral patterns of pleasure and mastery (Freud's "anal
stage"), makes it possible for a child to get involved with a
wider circle of parental persons (fathers, uncles and aunts,
helpers) who offer developmental support to and yet also
some (more or less) severe restraining of another basic
human strength—will. Indeed, the experiences of the second
stage of life remain basic as the first encounter (not *too*
inhibitive, one must hope) of willfulness with the shame and
self-doubt now readily aroused in the human being by punishment, shaming, and (yes) belittling. This continues for the

rest of life with every individual's continued protective and yet also restrictive regulation by the communal law and order within which the human being must, stage for stage, find a "rightful" place regulated by a systematic justice.

Now comes the play age, which suggests a vital and, indeed, imaginative initiative in the world of play-provoking materials as shared within the basic family—now including the siblings and "playmates" in the disciplined interplay with whom the growing being must learn creatively to exercise and yet also to limit (without too much of a sense of guilt or of inhibition) the hope of eventually realizing some purposeful anticipations within the social order of ideal and evil roles.

But then, in the school age, playmates become schoolmates, even as teachers are added to the ranks of parental authorities who represent and teach something of the basic competence that must eventually find its inventive function in the given work order with a technological order.

And then, again, comes that vast expansion of a hope for a more or less self-chosen identity called adolescence. Here our chart expands the radius of involvements to include peer groups and, especially, adult models, whether present and active among the young person's mentors or apparent on the horizon as heroes and leaders. A whole new world awaits the young person's development of a sense of reliable fidelity, which now calls for an ideological world view.

There follows young adulthood, first in the form of an involvement in freely chosen friendships, partnerships, and sexual relations, dominated as they now are by a sense and capacity for genitality, and yet also committed to a true sense of intimacy and love. At this stage, affiliative ritualizations find their up-to-date and appropriate versions in communal orders of affiliation, cooperation, and competition. While an absence of all such potential commitments can lead only to a sense of delinquency or, indeed, of isolation (sometimes an essential temporary step toward a true choice), a too elitistic group membership can lead to a more or less isolating exclusivity. All these potential dangers can eventually be overcome only by a decisive turn to generative adulthood, a state of body and mind, character and activity, which must eventually come to represent one's circumscribed chance not just to be actually (and that means activatedly and activatingly) at home in this life but also to make it a home for following generations.

Matured adulthood, then, means a set of vital involvements in life's generative activities. Psychosexual development, as most psychoanalytic theory emphasizes, should now, above all, culminate in mutual genital pleasure. In terms of the whole life cycle, however, it is clear that adult libido is destined to reach some maturity in a number of generative ways: from a sexual procreativity to the day's technological productivity and whatever patterns of creativity have developed in the individual and his or her times. Some such combination must assure the vitality of an order of care to those wide areas of adult involvements which, according to a Hindu expression, guarantee the "maintenance of the world." All this, in short, leads to a participation in areas of involvement in which one can learn to take care of what one truly cares for.

In the study of old people, then, we must pay attention to the interrelation not only of passing or, indeed, past abilities available for the now "grandparental" care of who and what has been generated. The question is what actuality and mutuality can continue to exist in anticipated involvements and in foreseeable disinvovlements, for the old-age strength of wisdom also demands a compliance with what may be called some truly involved disinvolvement—and all this within a communal order.

Wisdom, then, probably is truly involved disinvolvement. Otherwise, the remaining involvement is a continuation of care, as it has become focused on procreativity, and/or productivity, and/or creativity. But the new affiliation now offered is some kind of grandparenthood (to be discussed in the next chapter), which must remain loyal to a defined and planned role for old age within an order of wisdom.

Heightened awareness is, as we will now see, an essential aspect of involvement. Yet *awareness* happens to be a word as rarely used in psychological treatises as is the term *I*. Nonetheless, in the very discussion of communal involvement, we must briefly clarify the relation of the awareness and of *I* to such more common terms as *consciousness*—or *ego* and *self.* This also leads us to one of the greatest problems in English translation of some of Freud's basic terms, for there is a difference between what Freud calls *"becoming* conscious" *(Bewusstwerden)* and *"being* conscious" *(Bewusstsein),* which seems to refer to a more inclusive state of awareness. A similar and deeply related difference exists above all in Freud's use of the German word *Ich* and its everyday meaning of "I," which in translations usually appears as "ego" even as it may be endlessly discussed as "self." This becomes important when we must account for our use of the words *vital involvement* in our very title, for vital involvements, we believe, result, subjectively speaking, in a heightened awareness that can by no means necessarily be claimed by the usual "ego." This is all the more important to us since in old age a human being must not only confront nonbeing but also face the final maturation of what we may call an existential identity.

First, then, a brief discussion of the dimensions of the

sense of "I." Thoroughly objectified by the dictionaries (here we quote *March's Thesaurus*), *I,* of course, is simply the "self-designating pronoun" and thus, in all languages, the thinker and speaker as distinguished from everyone else. But then, *I* is also said to mean "the spiritual personality," which suggests an existential identity, while the *ego* is the "self considered as the seat of consciousness." All this leads one to continue to ponder the various meanings of *I.* *

The word *I,* then, in all languages, is the verbal assurance that each of us is a center of awareness in the center of the universe, and this with the sense of a coherent and continuous identity; in other words, we are alive and aware of it. (No wonder that, in order to grant such an experience to each other and to say "We" on a universal level, we may need a faith such as Moses taught when he claimed that on asking Him who He was, God replied, "I AM THAT I AM.")

In the end, therefore, when we speak of "I" as something we sense even as we say it, it seems to express an awareness, or a need for an awareness, approximated by a list of adjectives like these:

> central rather than peripheral in space and time
> luminous rather than overshadowed
> active and activated rather than passive
> continuous rather than scattered
> indivisible rather than divided
> inclusive rather than isolated and excluded
> safely bounded rather than invaded or evading
> chosen rather than bypassed
> etc.

It will be clear that all of these dimensions, though "at issue" throughout all the stages of life, are all at specific risk

---

*In *Identity: Youth and Crisis* (New York: W. W. Norton, 1968).

in old age, that "last" stage in which the senses and, with them, all space and time connections are destined to lose more or less inevitably some of their power of coherence— even as one knows that physical existence itself is coming to an end. All this makes for a number of specific dystonic and antipathic trends, listed on Chart 2, such as despair, (self-) disdain, and general dogmatism.

But it must be equally clear that the sense of "I," in old age, still has a once-for-all chance of transcending time-bound identities and sensing, if only in the simplest terms, an all-human and existential identity like that which the world religions and ideologies have attempted to create—if not without the hazard, sooner or later, of becoming themselves militant dogmas.

But lest the term *sense of I* and the adjectives descriptive of it still seem to suggest a dominant self-centeredness, let us reiterate the two essential qualities we claimed must characterize a *vital* involvement: actuality and mutuality. The prerequisite descriptive clauses just listed will, we hope, suggest a sense of reality that is an active and, in fact, an interactive involvement within a communal "actuality," and a shared sense of "we" within a communal mutuality.

All in all, in old age, many of the developmental concerns of earlier and earliest stages are being refaced, as the then-acquired capacities, traits, and involvements are now undergoing some disdevelopment.

II

The Voices of
Our Informants

I. INTEGRITY AND DESPAIR: WISDOM

This section explores the eight psychosocial themes as they seem to "come to word" in the lifelong experiences, observations, and insights offered by the elders who took part in our study. As we have explained, each stage in the life cycle involves the individual in reintegrating, in new, age-appropriate ways, those psychosocial themes that were ascendant in earlier periods. At every stage, the individual incorporates these earlier themes in the process of bringing into balance the tension that is now focal. Ranging in age from the early seventies through the late nineties, our informants may all be viewed as moving through the stage of life we refer to as old age. Thus, they may be understood as seeking to bring into balance the tension between a sense of integrity, of enduring comprehensiveness, and an opposing sense of despair, of dread and hopelessness. In addition, these elders are, through a complex of processes that are partly conscious and partly unconscious, attempting to reconcile the earlier psy-chosocial themes (generativity and stagnation, intimacy and isolation, identity and identity confusion, and so on) and to integrate them in relation to current, old-age development.

But what are the activities, the concerns, the involvements through which our informants engage in these processes? What are the terms in which they reexperience the eight different themes that we identify as the psychosocial tensions of a lifetime? How, on the basis of a unique life cycle and a unique complex of psychosocial dynamics, does each individual struggle to reconcile earlier themes in order to bring into balance a lifelong sense of trustworthy wholeness and an opposing sense of bleak fragmentation? What experiences and societal circumstances do these people share, as simple concomitants of being old at the same time and in the same place, and, perhaps, as a result of having been young under similarly common conditions? How is it that one individual may seem able to integrate painful conditions of old age into a new form of psychosocial strength, while another may respond to similar conditions in a fashion that seems to inhibit effective integration and healthy, ongoing develop-ment?

The chapters that follow explore our informants' descrip-tions of and reflections on their own lives, as we attempt to begin to answer some of these questions. Beginning with old age's tension between integrity and despair, we will move back through all of the earlier psychosocial themes. We will consider various ways that elders' efforts to make of the entire life cycle a unified whole lead them to struggle to bring each psychosocial theme into such balance as may be possi-ble.

It is through this last stage that the life cycle weaves back on itself in its entirety, ultimately integrating maturing forms of hope, will, purpose, competence, fidelity, love, and care, into a comprehensive sense of wisdom. Throughout life, the individual has, on some level, anticipated the finality of old age, experiencing an existential dread of "not-being" alongside an ever-present process of integrating those behaviors and restraints, those choices and rejections, those essential strengths and weaknesses over time that constitute what we have called the sense of "I" in the world. In old age this tension reaches its ascendancy. The elder is challenged to draw on a life cycle that is far more nearly completed than yet to be lived, to consolidate a sense of wisdom with which to live out the future, to place him- or herself in perspective among those generations now living, and to accept his or her place in an infinite historical progression.

Burdened by physical limitations and confronting a personal future that may seem more inescapably finite than ever before, those nearing the end of the life cycle find themselves struggling to accept the inalterability of the past and the unknowability of the future, to acknowledge possible mistakes and omissions, and to balance consequent despair with the sense of overall integrity that is essential to carrying on. For perhaps the first time, they find themselves recognizing that death may well come sooner rather than later. With their special perspective on the life cycle, these individuals are in a position to serve as guides for the futures of those who follow, at the same time that they must struggle to find guides on whom they can rely in considering their own futures and that of our world as a whole.

In earlier years, several of our informants anticipated life in old age through their relationships with grandparents and other old people they admired. Now, finally old themselves, they look for guidance back to the elders they have held in highest regard from their earliest years. One woman cites the sense of humor displayed so abundantly by both of her grandmothers. She says she has tried to be old with such a sense of humor, and she hopes to be remembered for "having humor, like my grannies." Another recalls her grandmother's final years: "I used to take care of her the last years of her life, when she was senile and got lost. She was so cute, and I never really thought of her as being old—just as needing help." This woman has close relationships with all of her grandchildren. She speaks warmly and lovingly of the paths they are following with their lives, and her comments suggest that they think of her often and with great fondness and affection. Her comments do not indicate that the grandchildren think of her as old. Rather, they seem to reflect her view of herself as she relates to them—always interested, concerned, and eager to be supportive. In fact, this woman can be somewhat territorial. She is also quite set in her ways. But from these rather unassailable positions she is always available for a visit or a telephone conversation, always reliable as a cheering section. She certainly conveys an assurance that, should she ever require the kind of care her grandmother needed, her grandchildren would try to respond with the same loving helpfulness that she recalls from her own grandchildhood.

For some elders, parents, rather than grandparents, served as early models for old age. Several of our informants cite parental wisdom and good judgment as the qualities they most respect and as those they most fervently hope they themselves demonstrate. One woman now sees in her parents admirable qualities to which she did not pay adequate attention in earlier life: "Mother was very wise in her way. She was strict and she demanded respect, but she'd do anything for us that she could. Father always cheered us on and bragged about us." In recent years, all of her children have been involved in divorces and struggles over child custody. As they have come to her, she has tried more consciously than ever before to demonstrate these qualities she recalls from her parents—to be wise, to be strict, and to be a source of support and encouragement. In earlier years, our subject experienced Mother's strictness in painful conflict with Father's overt supportiveness and encouragement. Now she is coming to reconcile these apparent opposites. For perhaps the first time in her life, she has found herself beginning to understand the wisdom necessary to being empathic while not condoning selfishness, being helpful while not intrusive, being proud while not smug. And she sees the roots of this wisdom in the parents of her childhood.

Another woman tells an anecdote about her mother, illustrating both her own philosophy of old age and the source of that philosophy: "My mother was eighty years old and plants an apple tree and says, 'In five years we'll have apples.'" This woman, now in her eighties herself, has always believed in living each day to its fullest, without worry about what may or may not be possible tomorrow. Where other elders participate in activities on a day-to-day basis, uncertain of or unwilling to count on the future, she continues to behave in a fashion that takes a future for granted. For example, she has recently enrolled in a community college course in sign language. It seems that the college required an enrollment of fifteen students, and a neighbor with a deaf relative persuaded her to become the fifteenth. Initially, she enrolled only as a favor to her neighbor. But now she has become an enthusiast and explains, "In a few more semesters I'll be fluent. Then I'll be able to go to the museum and persuade them to provide tours in sign, for deaf art lovers."

Other informants look to their contemporaries—some to media personalities and some to local friends or relatives—

as guides along what they regard as the path of successful aging. One man points to Bob Hope with respect and admiration: "He has amassed a fortune. He married and stayed with the same wife for many years. He has been wonderfully unselfish in his trips to Vietnam. We are nearly the same age, and I look to his life as a standard for my own." A woman points to a neighbor, a tiny little woman who makes cookies for her friends and takes them around as an excuse to check up on everyone. This neighbor stopped by during one of our interviews, bustling in and out and leaving the apartment filled with a nearly palpable cheerfulness. After her friend's departure, our informant pointed out, "She has had two hip operations, but you can't even tell that her walk is funny unless you know to look for it. She had two falls, one on each hip, and if she drops something on the floor it is very difficult for her to pick it up. But she trots around and does things, giving tours and such! Now, how could I worry about my own aches or pains when I always have a box of her cookies, staring me in the face?"

A third individual points to a man in his local senior center: "He is well liked by the people around here, and he's accomplished, and he still has a very good attitude about him and toward people. He came by and plowed that area for me. He'd just plowed for himself and for some widow lady on the other side of the hill there, and so he plowed for me too." This aging Good Samaritan is far from healthy. He has apparently undergone such extensive digestive-tract surgery that "inside him, he has more nylon than flesh and blood." To our informant, he represents both a relentless unwillingness to give in and a boundless source of consideration for friends and neighbors. In his own life, our informant strives to live out these same qualities, helping neighbors with chores at which he is competent, ingeniously sharing those of his possessions that he feels will give pleasure to others, and trying, always, to use his energies in a way that will leave other people glad he lives nearby. For all of these individuals, the qualities they note in the people they identify as valued elders, from the past and in the present, are qualities they try to demonstrate in their own old age. Striving to emulate such ideals seems to give them a kind of strength, to counterbalance old age's uncertainty about how to behave now, in order to be true to the past as well as to prepare for what may come next.

Most of our elders are able to discuss differences they notice in themselves and their friends as old people, in comparison with what they remember from younger days. For many, these changes include a kind of increased concern for and tolerance of the world and its multifarious inhabitants. These people describe both themselves and their aged contemporaries as more tolerant, more patient, more open-minded, more understanding, more compassionate, and less critical than they were in younger years. In a variety of ways, many agree that "patience is one thing you know better when you're old than when you were young." "Old people are slower to anger . . . with people who don't understand their point of view. They are able to take the vicissitudes of life in a calmer manner." "Nothing shocks me any more." "Now I can see both sides."

Many of our informants seem to be open to considerations they used to view as incompatible. They also seem to express a new concern for issues they previously all but ignored. For example, for one lifelong liberal activist, the newly developed ability to "see both sides" involves the later-life moderation of her liberal political ideals, in a movement toward conservatism. Lifelong conservatives who experience themselves as increasingly tolerant and patient seem to notice a corresponding movement toward liberalism. This notion of seeing both sides is closely related to the old-age process of reconciling one's relationship to the plethora of people and values with whom one has coexisted over the course of a lifetime. In later life, the accustomed imperative of maintenance activity—middle age's pressure to take definite action in order to maintain responsibility for family, institution, and community—seems to give way to the faculty of entertaining a variety of points of view.

Not all of the elders in our study describe themselves or their contemporaries wholly as increasingly open-minded or tolerant. Many make the opposite observation that "old people get more set in their ways." And several, caught in apparent internal contradiction, claim to notice both phenomena in themselves. Perhaps this contradiction is more apparent than real. Perhaps being set in one's own ways is not incompatible with tolerating other people's points of view. In fact, an increasing integration of one's own style perhaps permits a new understanding of others' preferences for *their* own styles.

A number of our informants discuss their own old age in the context of friends and neighbors who are also aging. Some allude to loneliness and to speculations about being missed when they themselves die. They look around old neighborhoods and senior centers, and they sigh, "I'm sorry these people are aging, because one by one they are leaving us." Others seem to take comfort in the fact that they are not aging alone. One of these recalls, "When we moved in here forty years ago, we were [all] young, and the neighbors have all grown old with us." Others note the aging of friends and neighbors almost as a way to avoid acknowledging such processes in themselves. Of these, one admits, "I never expected to get old. Others, but not me." Observing and reacting to the aging of their contemporaries seems to help these people to integrate aspects of their own aging, to view their individual experiences in a reassuring social perspective. For all its frightening concomitants—recognized and unrecognized—growing old, in these terms, is a powerful confirmation of membership in a human race that is more expansive and more enduring than any one lifetime.

In order to avoid succumbing to deterioration and depression, several of the elders in our study have developed philosophies of aging that espouse a determination "to keep old age licked." On the basis of ongoing involvement with various aspects of the world, one man pragmatically asserts, "If you're going to keep on living, you better keep on growing." Some individuals describe energetic commitment to a daily routine. One woman says, "I can't wait to get into bed at night with a good book. I can't wait to get up in the morning and have a cup of coffee. That's my life." Others remain actively involved with people, declaring, "I just keep busy doing things that I like to do, and things for other people. . . . Once in a while I get a little pain, but it doesn't stop me from going and doing things." Still others stop short of describing their personal strategies for aging with integrity; they seem to prefer, instead, to make prescriptions for the elderly in general: "Old people think too much about dying, feeling ill and neglected. They need to be needed. Doing volunteer work would solve the problem for everyone."

Most of our informants seem to find themselves, almost involuntarily, thinking about dying and about feeling ill, depressed, and somehow let down. To some extent, these thoughts are integral to old age in our society, reflecting a desperation that confronts all elders. However, most people struggle to counterbalance these associations with thoughts of more optimistic, life-affirming involvement. It is almost as though they believe that feelings of pessimism, discouragement, and simple exhaustion must be all but excluded from conversation, lest they jeopardize fragile tendencies toward energetic optimism.

The following ninety-year-old is one of very few elders in our study who choose to mention regret at having lived so long and readiness to die. He observes, "You have had your life and lived a long time. You know the saying, 'The good die young.' Well, I must have been terribly bad in my youth, because I am still living." He does not make this comment in jest. Although he is not ill, he is weak enough that walking down the block threatens to consume nearly a whole hour and a whole afternoon's energy. He is still interested in politics and literature, but the direct objects of his life's passions are inaccessible and sadly missed. A bit unsteadily, he goes on, "When you get to my age, why, I am willing to die any time. The only thing that keeps me alive is my obligation to the family." For this man, feelings of later-life responsibility to family members conflict with the readiness, and perhaps eagerness, to die that also seems to be a part of his integrity in old age. Where other, often younger, subjects emphasize the need of the aged to be needed, this very old man now perhaps feels more burdened than gratified by being needed in such a way. His conflict reminds us that death has its place in the life cycle. The task of the elder is not simply to reaffirm life, to reinforce psychosocial strengths by maintaining meaningful involvement with people and activities. The task of the elder also includes coming to accept the inevitability of death's enforced leave-taking.

Throughout the life cycle, anticipating and planning for the future represents a kind of psychological preparation for the years of life that are expected yet to come. Although an individual life may be cut short at any moment, in childhood, youth, and middle age the normative expectation is of a personal future that will last for decades. In old age, however, the duration of the future is far more uncertain. Earlier life's illusions of unlimited time are buffeted by the swelling certitude of mortality. Still, as part of life itself, our informants think about their futures. Many speak in terms of a direct continuation of the lives they have always lived, that is, of daily activities and, for some, of longer-range plans. One speaks of continuing to work out issues of household responsibility with a partner. One talks of recovering from a medical condition so that he can resume eating tasty foods. Several plan to continue work on written autobiographies. Some resolve to get more regular exercise and to develop new avocational interests. One hopes to straighten out previously difficult relationships with children. Some anticipate beginning to relax from the rigid work schedules to which they have adhered for the past sixty years. At least to some extent, these people view the future as a time for activity. It may provide an opportunity to do things for which there has never before been time. It may be a time to continue to enjoy those activities that have long been sources of pleasure. It may also offer the chance to make amends, in the present, for misunderstandings of the past.

For perhaps all of our informants, the notion of a personal future is openly and directly tied to the recognition that death may well not be far off. Those cited above view the time that remains as a valuable resource, to be used well for as long as it lasts. One explains, "I don't think I'll be here in ten or fifteen years. That's why I love . . . to do things now." In a less concrete way, others view continuing to live as long as possible as a goal in itself. They may set milestones for themselves. Several people in their eighties hope to live to be ninety; one woman adds the wish to be a blond ninety-year-old. These people do not seem to equate their time alive with opportunity for specific accomplishments. Rather, remaining alive represents an accomplishment in and of itself. For many, it seems to be the only goal they still feel able to pursue.

In the face of death's probable imminence, many of our subjects find the future difficult to plan for. "You don't know whether you are going to be here tomorrow or not," notes one of them. "Nobody does, of course, but when you are older your chances are more questionable." After a lifetime of planning, of sacrificing today's pleasures for tomorrow's anticipated rewards, they struggle to accept the realistic uncertainty that makes this lifelong behavior pattern suddenly inappropriate. The painfulness of this unfamiliar incertitude is suggested by the extent to which many of them, unasked, assert that they do not worry. Some do not worry about how much longer they will live. Other do not worry about where they will live out the future that remains. Others do not worry about the future at all, preferring to let it take care of itself. Quite realistically, these elders view the personal future as far more doubtful and unknowable at this stage of life than it ever seemed before. To many, though, wondering about these unknowns seems to be inseparable from worrying, which seems, in turn, to be inseparable from overwhelming despair. In an attempt to come to terms with this ultimate mystery, they find themselves struggling to ignore it altogether.

Although many of our informants profess not to worry about future life, they cannot hide their fear of the death that will follow. One says tremblingly, "On New Year's night, when they drop that ball, I am so glad I lived another year. I don't like to die at all! I am frightfully afraid of death!" To some, death looms as a painful, lingering process they are prepared to bargain to avoid. One individual explains tearfully, "I don't want to get into pain, and I am starting to get it. I have no qualms about dying, but I don't want to suffer." Others associate death with a loneliness and abandonment that they discuss only indirectly. Many assert quite honestly that they do not want to be a burden to anyone else. What most do not openly articulate is the desperate hope that if they cannot avoid becoming a burden, someone will be willing to accept responsibility for their care.

As our subjects near the end of the life cycle, many begin to see their grandchildren as extensions of themselves into the indefinite future. One explains, "I do not have *personal* thoughts about the future, but I do think about my grandchildren's futures." Some cite particular grandchildren with whom they identify for reasons as diverse as eye color, facial expression, similarity in name, and shared personality traits. This concern for the grandchildren's futures enables them to move beyond the inescapability and unknowability of their own death, to a concern for the long lives that they see ahead of these young people. And this personal concern for the well-being of the grandchildren is but one facet of these elders' concern for the future well-being of the world as a whole.

When our informants are asked to discuss the future, their comments move quickly to a concern about a disturbing present and a sense of societal, and even worldwide, drift about which they are none too sanguine. Many of them seem to subscribe to the overall evaluations "Things are terrible in the world today" and "There is nothing I can do personally." Although the criteria for these assessments may vary from person to person, the assessments themselves are strikingly, and chillingly, uniform: "I'm glad I'm not young and facing

a future in the world today." "I'm glad I won't have to live
in the world the children are inheriting." "I sometimes worry
about the future of the planet, and I am sort of glad we have
done all we have done. I don't know if the future is going to
be as good as the past." "As things are developing, I doubt
if I would want to bring children into the world today."

Each individual regards different aspects of today's world
as critical. Some mention world politics—specifically, their
concern that the United States must avoid being taken over
by the Soviet Union. Some point to ecology, feeling that the
planet is losing its ability to provide for human beings and
that conservation for the future is our duty. Many list perceived ills in American society. In citing issues like greed at
the individual, industrial, and national levels; lack of respect
for traditional American ideals; and the absence of commitment, loyalty, and conviction in family, interpersonal, and
institutional relationships, these elders are identifying areas
in which they feel society is going in the wrong direction and
for which they think they know a better direction. However,
they also recognize that despite their unique perspective and
insight, they do not have the power to implement their
suggestions. Several conclude, "There's no use worrying
when there's nothing you can do, but I do have thoughts. I
am certainly concerned."

As our informants wondered aloud what kind of world
their grandchildren would occupy, we spoke with them of
the possibility of nuclear war. Some profess an almost frantic
confidence in mankind's ability to avoid such a confrontation: "No one would dare start it." "I can't conceive of
anybody setting off the first blast." "I hope we'll have safeguards enough to avoid disaster." "I have confidence." "I'm
not alarmed." "People will be judicious. Probably." "I think
mankind is sensible enough to realize nuclear warfare can't

happen. They'll be strong enough not to let it be accidental." Perhaps these people really do have faith that, either by divine plan or by human restraint, a nuclear catastrophe will be avoided. Perhaps, however, more than real confidence, these assertions represent attempts to avoid the despair that would almost certainly be overwhelming at the full recognition, on the part of each of these elders, not just that his or her own life will soon end but that the whole world as he or she has known it may be about to come to an end as well.

Other individuals defend against despair by seeking to be optimistic about the consequences of nuclear war: "I doubt if it would eliminate the world population. It would set us back hundreds of years." "If things get out of hand, maybe it is a good thing to stop and start over. Turn the pages back a hundred years and start over." But such optimism sounds as desperately hollow as the confidence noted above. Our informants cannot point to any basis more convincing than personal fervor for the faith that humankind will survive what they seem to identify as our impatient, narrow selfishness coupled with an advanced technological ability to destroy ourselves. Rather, they seem to speculate about humankind's surviving a nuclear holocaust primarily in order to handle their own feelings. Only a very few speak openly of the prospect that "we'll *all* be blown up. . . . Fighting before was one thing, but this is terrible! If one of these things is dropped, everybody is going to be killed, and who is going to be left to do anything?"

These elders do not prescribe a worldwide strategy for avoiding nuclear destruction. Instead, they focus on smaller issues, voicing clear ideas about how individual human beings should live—as long as we have the privilege of living at all: "You have to be tolerant and respect other people's judgments." "Respect and kindness are essential. . . . And patience. . . . If you learn to wait, you appreciate the things you've wanted for a long time far more." "We have to think more of the other fellow. Set an example and offer real help." "Parents should pay more attention to their children. Be consistent. Use discipline." "You have to believe in a here-after, and a God. Something bigger than you are." "We can only do the best we can. Love your neighbor as yourself. Make the world a better place." These prescriptions are offered by our informants to those who will survive them. By and large, they also closely resemble the prescriptions these elders might have received from their own parents or grand-parents. They are the principles according to which these people have tried to live their lives, and according to which they now take stock of their pasts, in an effort to move into the future with mature wisdom.

As our informants distill from the past that which they view as essential to the future, many turn to religion—to current beliefs and to those of a lifetime. For these people, religion has been a force around which life's decisions have been made and actions been taken, through all stages. Now, as they look to a future that may seem more frightening and unknowable than ever before, lifelong religious faith offers a kind of consolation. One woman finds herself recalling a rhyming version of the Ten Commandments that she learned as a child. Another thinks often of the weekly services she attended as a little girl, proudly wearing her Sunday best and tightly holding on to her mother's hand. In later life, both of these women seem to be invoking childhood religious expression as a source of current religious strength and inte-gration, in the face of inevitable despair.

Some of our subjects seem to find welcome reassurance in the notion of ritual church attendance. The woman men-tioned immediately above draws on her childhood for this ritualized experience, noting that in recent years she feels an increasing need to return to this earlier practice and the sense of comfort it offered. Others of our elders speak of the importance of going to church, whether or not they actually attend. Perhaps the very thought of this ritualized community behavior allows the reconciling of a lifetime of faith with an unfamiliar desperation. Perhaps, too, it reflects a sense of the integrity of the life cycle, the generational cycle, and a larger cycle of community.

At the start of this section, we noted that the process of bringing into balance feelings of integrity and despair involves a review of and a coming to terms with the life one has lived thus far. An important component of this process is the acknowledging and accepting of past choices, made along life's course. Many of the elders in our study look back now, quite satisfied with how they have chosen to live their lives—with the people they married, with the ways they raised their children, with the kinds of work they did. Generally, these people conclude, "There are no regrets that I know of for things that have happened or that I've done." We must note that this currently expressed satisfaction does not necessarily imply lifelong contentment. In fact, historical data indicate that in earlier life a number of these same individuals experienced periods of profound unhappiness and restlessness, which they attributed to misguided decisions concerning spouse, career, child rearing, or living arrangements.

Why do so many of our informants refrain from mentioning earlier discontent? What do these omissions suggest about the old-age struggle to bring a sense of integrity into scale with a sense of despair? Perhaps these people are engaging in the process of "pseudo-integration," of constructing a satisfactory overall view of the life cycle by denying those elements they find to be unacceptable. Perhaps, more consciously, they are choosing to maintain a measure of privacy in interviews with researchers who, however sympathetic, are known scarcely more intimately than strangers. Perhaps, as well, these omissions reflect a lifelong process of reintegration and recasting, whereby events and circumstances that were once experienced as painful have, over the years, taken on new meanings as part of the whole life cycle. Perhaps, in addition, they indicate that over the years traumatic events have been put into perspective.

Another component of the reviewing and accepting of life already lived has to do with the inalterability of the past. As with the issue of early choices, some elders express unmitigated, lifelong satisfaction in exclamations like the following: "I must have been born under a lucky star. During my entire lifetime I never really had a disappointment." Others acknowledge that the path was not always smooth, and that they were not always able to meet unexpected demands in an appropriate fashion or to handle unforeseen emergencies in a manner that had the desired consequences. All are struggling somehow to accept the notion that, whether or not they could have behaved differently in the past, they cannot *now* alter decisions made or courses of action taken *then*. In particular, several of our informants look back on their earlier-life powerlessness to keep a loved one from death. They wonder, "Why wasn't there something we could have done?" They simply cannot absolve themselves of responsibility for the death of a spouse or a child, and they ruminate endlessly. Should they have consulted another doctor? Weren't there signs or symptoms they could have seen earlier if they had only looked carefully enough? Wasn't there some additional measure of care they could have provided that might have saved or, at least, prolonged life? But these painful ruminations come into balance with a recognition that nothing can now be done to change the emergencies, the responses, and the consequences of those long-past events.

As the elder seeks to consolidate a sense of lifelong wisdom and perspective, he or she endeavors, ideally, not to exclude legitimate feelings of cynicism and hopelessness, but to admit them in dynamic balance with feelings of human wholeness. Later life brings many, quite realistic reasons for experiencing despair: aspects of a past we fervently wish had been different; aspects of a present that cause unremitting pain; aspects of a future that are uncertain and frightening. And, of course, there remains inescapable death, that one aspect of the future which is both wholly certain and wholly unknowable. Thus, some despair must be acknowledged and integrated as a component of old age, anticipated from the beginning of life. The elder engages in this integration as he or she acts and reflects on the various issues discussed above. In addition, this ultimate integration comprises all of those conscious and unconscious processes by which the individual at the end of life seeks to reexperience and to bring again into scale each of the psychosocial themes that have, in turn, given shape to the life cycle and that we will explain, stage by stage, in the pages that follow.

Not all of our informants are fully able to use—as a source of comfort, understanding, or compassion—the perspective afforded by a long life. Nor do they all succeed in demonstrating, in their own old age, the qualities they admire in valued elders. However, all of these people are struggling to bring lifelong dystonic tendencies into balance with acknowledged psychosocial strengths. For some, too, weaknesses continue to outweigh strengths in ways that remain quite painful. We shall illustrate some of these conflicts in subsequent chapters. At this point, we must emphasize that, regardless of what may appear to be individual success or failure in reexperiencing the psychosocial themes of a lifetime, our elders are all involved in the process of trying. It is this effort that is the basis for growth at all stages of the life cycle.

2. GENERATIVITY AND STAGNATION: CARE

The experiences of caring, nurturing, and maintaining—which are the essence of generativity—make of the stages of life a life *cycle,* re-creating the beginnings of the cycle in each newborn. These same experiences make of the sequence of life cycles a *generational* cycle, irrevocably binding each generation to those that gave it life and to those for whose life it is responsible. Thus, reconciling lifelong generativity and stagnation involves the elder in a review of his or her own years of active responsibility for nurturing the next generations, and also in an integration of earlier-life experiences of caring and of self-concern in relation to previous generations. That is, today's elder must balance the feelings of generativity and stagnation developed in the course of middle age's active parenting, working, and creating, all completed decades before. In addition, the elder must come to terms with the caring and the lack of caring experienced as a child, at the hands of his or her own parents, and as an adult, having been responsible for these same parents in their old age.

We understand middle adulthood's generative responsibility for the "maintenance of the world" in terms of the interrelated realms of people, products, and ideals. It is therefore the responsibility of each generation of adults to bear, nurture, and guide those people who will succeed them as adults, as well as to develop and maintain those societal institutions and natural resources without which successive generations will not be able to survive. Giving up the official positions of responsibility in the family and community may confront the elder with unwelcome feelings of stagnation, as clearly defined demands for generativity decrease and accustomed generative activity becomes inappropriate. In addition, diminishing energy and physical capacities may place undeniable limits on the earlier-life behaviors related to caring for a family, a profession, or an institution. However, as we will note in considering each psychosocial theme at the end of life, old age may impose its own, unique demands, and it may offer its own, unique opportunities, for integrating inevitable stagnation with new and modified involvement in the lifelong capacity for generative caring.

The reconciling of generativity and stagnation involves the elder in expressing a "grand-generativity" that is somehow beyond middle age's direct responsibility for maintaining the world. The roles of aging parent, grandparent, old friend, consultant, adviser, and mentor all provide the aging adult with essential social opportunities to experience grand-generativity in current relationships with people of all ages. In these relationships, the individual seeks to integrate outward-looking care for others with inward-looking concern for self. As a complement to caring for others, the elder is also challenged to accept from others that caring which is required, and to do so in a way that is itself caring. In the context of the generational cycle, it is incumbent upon the aged to enhance feelings of generativity in their care givers from the younger generations.

The capacity for grand-generativity incorporates care for the present with concern for the future—for today's younger generations in their futures, for generations not yet born, and for the survival of the world as a whole. It contributes to the sense of immortality that becomes so important in the individual's struggle to transcend realistic despair as the end of life approaches, inevitably. However, grand-generative concern for the future in the abstract must be integrated with simple, direct caring for the specific individuals who are part of life today. The elder who is preoccupied with concern for the world's infinite unknowability runs the very real risk of wounding, through neglect or inadvertent action, familiar individuals—relatives, colleagues, friends, and caretakers— with whom contact is most immediate and with whom personal concern is likely to be mutually greatest.

Despite the multiple facets of overall generativity noted above, among most of our subjects, concern for their children dominates both their reflections on earlier life's guidance and nurturance and their current involvements in caring. For most of these people, it seems that parenthood has been the primary focus of adulthood responsibility. It is not surprising, therefore, that it is through reconsidering their children's adulthood successes and failures that they seek, retroactively, to validate the responsible caring they themselves provided in their years of active parenting.

Most of our informants, like parents at any age, are eager to voice pride in their children's accomplishments. "My sons are all very rich men." "My kids all grew up staunch and sturdy, and have such good characters." "They turned out real smart. They all went to college." In old age, these people seem to feel that their parenting of twenty to sixty years ago is responsible for the successful people their children are today. One woman was quoted, throughout her active parenting years, as bemoaning the social inequities between those who had money and those, like the members of her family, who did not. She has always loudly protested that "money is no measure of a man," and she is quick to cite newspaper reports to foolish statements made or illegal actions committed by people of means. Still, the extent to which themes of insufficient money, unfair pricing of essential goods, and advantage taken of impecunious people dominate her conversation suggests that this issue is central to her view of success. Like her father, her husband worked hard for relatively meager financial rewards. Consequently, as a daughter and then as a wife and mother, she also remained without wealth. Today she is extraordinarily proud that each of her children owns and runs an extremely profitable manufacturing business. Although she herself could never climb the ladder of financial success, she is proud to have raised her children in such a way that they are now able to give *their* children the best of everything.

In addition to noting overall success, elders consider their children's parenting as a supplementary way to review their own active parenting of an earlier decade. Many people praise aspects of the children's parenting that are meaningful to them. Some seek to validate their own emphasis on and achievements in these same areas. One lifelong homemaker admires the way her youngest daughter runs a busy household and manages a large family. This woman is proud of her husband's affectionate observation, fifty years earlier, that "Pearlie is a lousy bookkeeper, but you'll never find a wife or mother to match her." She was successful at what was important (that is, pleasing her husand and raising her children), and that was all that really mattered. In the intervening decades, our society's expectations have shifted so that it is no longer taken absolutely for granted, as it was during this woman's young motherhood, that home and family are the only important domains for a woman's generative energies. However, today this subject does not speak of a family emphasis on the grandchildren's academic or athletic achievements. She does not mention her daughter's level of education or possible interest in working outside the home. These aspects of her daughter's family life are not particularly meaningful to her, and she simply does not bring them up. What she highlights is the fact that she has raised a daughter who is successful at what Mother regards as important. In living out this success, the daughter is both vindicating her mother's sense of values and confirming her effectiveness in transmitting them.

Our informants find it important to view themselves as having been good parents—as having provided their children the wherewithal to succeed professionally, to raise and guide yet another generation, and to surmount with integrity whatever adversity they may confront. Thus, they are able, at least in retrospect, to find silver linings in many of the storm clouds the children have weathered. For example, one woman describes her younger daughter as having led a life of disjunctions. Despite an excellent academic record at a prestigious university, she left college to marry her high school sweetheart and become the mother of six children. She divorced her husband when he refused to terminate a long-term love affair with another woman. For several years, she supported herself and the children by doing substitute teaching, and then by founding and running a successful tutoring agency. She has always pursued sculpture as a hobby. Now that her children are grown, she has left her company and sold her house, to devote all of her time to her sculpture. Over the years, our informant was upset and worried at each one of her daughter's changes of life course.

The informant had herself left college to get married, and she has always regretted her failure to complete her own degree. From an early age, the daughter was a better student than her mother had ever been. Our informant was both proud of this academic excellence and relieved that it apparently exonerated her for her own earlier decision. Although she had prematurely terminated her own education, she had obviously instilled in her children a drive for educational achievement. Thanks to her values and training, they would not make the same mistake she had made. The daughter's sudden shift in course challenged her mother's hard-won sense of vindication. Perhaps, after all, she had not equipped her children to do better than she had been able to do.

Our informant had participated in a strong, secure, stable marriage that endured until her husband died, shortly after his retirement. The daughter's divorce and the ways in which she subsequently earned a living indicated to her mother that she did not enjoy stability or security in any sphere of her life. Today, in old age, our informant does not dwell on her daughter's difficulties or on the disjunctions in her life. Instead, she expresses pride in her daughter's courage, energy, and ingenuity, explaining, "She's so bright. She has so many different kinds of ideas. I'm so proud of all the different kinds of things she's accomplished! I know I don't have to worry about her, because whatever happens, she is the kind of person who will be able to land on her feet."

In keeping with our subjects' desire to regard their children's lives as a validation of their own generativity, they speak with great satisfaction of the children's good marriages. Such discussion provides them an opportunity to reconsider their own earlier intimacy and isolation. It also allows them to confirm their effectiveness in raising children who are capable of the adulthood satisfaction and responsibility of marital mutuality. However, not all of the children are involved in marriages their parents regard as good or

stable. In fact, nearly half of our subjects have seen at least
one of their children go through at least one divorce. It is
therefore particularly striking that many discuss the children's painful marital discontinuities and difficulties in terms
that highlight strength or growth in their divorcing child and
that, once again, by implication, validate their own earlier
parental effectiveness. When a woman muses, "I never could
figure out how he picked girls. We thought that marriage was
a mistake from the beginning," she is tacitly commending
her son for recognizing his mistake and not letting it ruin the
rest of his life. When another observes, "Her husband was a
very difficult man. She just wouldn't take it any more," she
is proud that her daughter stopped letting herself be taken
advantage of. The man who is "glad they settled this thing
in a friendly way," not as he had advised him to do, is also
praising his son for behaving with maturity and integrity. In
addition, he seems proud that his son has displayed more
maturity than he himself was inclined to do. Another man
explains, "When his wife left, I don't know whether he was
more upset or we were. But after all, it seems to have been
for the best in the long run." This man is alluding to his relief
that he views his son's second marriage as far happier and
more supportive than the first.

Not all of the elders succeed in their efforts to experience
generative confirmation in their children's adult lives. The
father of a son who, as an adult, has left several marriages
and has never held a steady job, muses, "I wonder if my son
is worse off or not for anything I've done. He never complains. But things aren't quite right." In earlier years, this
father viewed his son's behavior as uniformly irreproachable.
It is perhaps a mark of later-life success at beginning to
reconsider his sense of procreative generativity that in old
age this man is able both to notice that something is wrong

with his son and to wonder whether he is in any way responsible.

In addition to reexperiencing their own parenting vicariously, by evaluating their children, our subjects face these issues directly, as they look back on various aspects of themselves as the parents of young children, fifty or sixty years ago. Many place their early parenthood in a generational context, reminiscing about the extent to which they consciously perpetuated or broke away from family parenting styles. Many of our now-aged parents had themselves been raised very strictly. Some consciously maintained this uncompromising style, and they explain, "Of course, I imitated my parents' expectations that children must toe the line a bit, no arguments tolerated." Others believed in moderation and social evolution, and they tried, without being unduly permissive, to be more lenient than family traditions dictated. Rather than carry on what they perceived as unsatisfactory generational patterns, these people sought to establish healthier patterns for their children to carry into the future. Some feel that they effectively developed their own disciplinary styles, observing, "We were strict with the children, but we felt that if you overdo this you spoil all their pleasures." Others are less satisfied, musing, "I was more lenient with my children than my mother was with me. Too lenient, as a matter of fact." Regardless of the success of these efforts, in later life our subjects express satisfaction for having tried. The considering of their own parenting in terms of generational family style involves not only their caring for the well-being of the next generation but also their respect and appreciation for the feelings and judgments of the preceding generation. These concerns are all part of the involvement with the generational cycle that is such an important part of renewing a sense of generativity in old age.

Another dimension of the review of procreativity has to do with the emotion with which early parenthood is recalled. Some people look back on this period as the happiest time of their lives; they retell favorite stories and recount their own involvement in such children's activities as scouting, PTA, Sunday school, music lessons, and sports. Such reminiscing seems to provide a valued opportunity to reexperience the joyful exhilaration of their own younger years, as they struggle to integrate a meaningful sense of lifelong caring. In contrast, other people recall early parenthood with anxiety and regret, trying to balance feelings of inadequacy with a sense of success. Some focus on incidents about which they have felt guilty for decades. One man accuses himself of negligence while teaching his son to work in the woodshop, resulting in permanent injury to the boy's hand. Perhaps he hopes that talking about his guilt will enable him to integrate this incident more effectively into his overall sense of his fatherhood. Several people point, somewhat uncomfortably, to specific things they would do differently if they were given a second opportunity to raise their children. Some would be more patient or less "demanding and perfectionistic." Others would spend more time parenting and less time working. Some cannot say exactly what they would do differently, but they feel that their children's problems indicate that they were somehow inadequate parents. All of these recollections represent elders' efforts to come to terms, once and for all, with a responsibility that dominated their lives for decades and continues to hover over them today.

For our subjects, as for many of their age-mates, procreativity has overridden productivity and creativity as the major lifelong expression of generativity. We must remember that these people were young parents during the Depression. The exigencies of war and serious economic pressure made it difficult or even impossible for many of them to pursue their own educational and professional goals while raising families. To some extent, then, these people have always viewed their parenting accomplishments as substitutes for, and perhaps expressions of, their own unfulfilled ambitions. To some extent, they have experienced their children's creative and productive accomplishments as a validation of their own unexpressed creativity and productivity. Women who regret having had to leave school or creative careers, in order to marry and raise children, and men who had to take low-level jobs instead of pursuing higher education all reconcile facets of their own generativity by taking overwhelming pride in their children's academic, artistic, intellectual, and professional accomplishments.

But this vicarious realization of unfulfilled personal dreams is not unambivalent. A frustrated musician observes about his son, "He got the degree in music that was never available to me. And a teaching credential as well. That boy makes a good living." This subject had been identified as an especially talented child and had always wanted to make music his livelihood. He was having difficulty with a music major in college when he was drafted for World War I, and in some ways he viewed military service as a welcome break from his academic troubles. After the war, he did not return to school. Rather, he demonstrated appropriate adulthood responsibility by marrying his sweetheart and finding a job to support the family they would soon have. For most of his career, he worked at writing and selling advertising jingles, always hoping that his musical talent would be recognized and that he would be "discovered." But his hopes were in vain. He subordinated his serious musical ambitions to the necessity of supporting his family, and, particularly after rejecting advertising in favor of a more lucrative form of sales, he succeeded at this procreative dimension of generativity. Circumstances that were first societal and then economic led this man to abandon his efforts to actualize his own aspirations toward generative creativity. That these aspirations were complicated by early academic difficulties only intensifies the feelings of frustration and stagnation that he has carried with him, at having subordinated personal creativity to interpersonal procreativity. Over the years, he has been both proud and envious of his children's achievements in the arts.

Now nearly ninety, he takes less ambivalent pride in the children. No longer obliged to work each day to earn a living, he finds time to play his saxophone, to perform in the senior center, and to write entertaining songs about characters he has known over the years. Finally, he is actively engaged in nurturing his own creativity. A pervasive sense of stagnation in this realm need no longer interfere with his legitimate feelings of procreative generativity, at having supported a large family, helped his wife raise their children, and ensured that he and his wife will be adequately cared for throughout their old age.

An additional element of vicarious fulfillment through their children involves older people in seeing aspects of themselves, their partners, and their parents in the next generations. Our subjects are delighted to identify their own characteristics, interests, and talents in their children and grandchildren: "My son is a perfectionist, like me." "The kids are innately smart, like their father." "She has her mother's fire, that first girl of ours. She has more energy and more projects than anyone. Come to think of it, my mother had that fire, too. And my wife's two grandmothers." In seeking to identify family characteristics across several generations, these elders place themselves, as well as their children, in a continuity of generational history. The establishing of the next generations has to do in part with appropriately rooting them in their generational past. In so doing, older people may secure their own places, too, in the cycle of generations.

In old age's final reworking of issues of lifelong nurturance and concern, older people must come to terms with the earlier-life choices they made about how to express generativity and how, for whatever reasons, *not* to express it. As we have noted, these earlier choices most often emphasized caring for their children's long-range well-being over caring for themselves and their own talents and ambitions. In and of themselves, these procreative choices involved our subjects in integrating the ways they themselves had been cared for, and not cared for, in their own childhood. At the end of life, when they recognize that time to nurture their early-subordinated, long-stagnant interests is running out, several of our subjects are having difficulty coming to terms with the ways they have not expressed the creativity and productivity that also constitute a sense of caring. Some, like the musician discussed earlier, are taking advantage of the free time and diminished responsibilities of old age to develop creative and productive interests that have been dormant, often since late adolescence. Others, however, find themselves unable to take advantage of these later-life opportunities, and they experience some sense of stagnation.

One woman was an art student in her youth. Delicate and lovely herself, she painted small, pastel watercolors and produced intricate line drawings of fairy-tale images. This woman married young, and she and her husband worked in a family wholesale business that they founded together as a means of supporting the children. The family was plagued by illness and emotional difficulties. The business absorbed all the effort they could muster, but it never seemed to find a solid financial footing. These people were not particularly interested in wholesaling per se. They chose it originally as likely to provide a stable income for the family. Over the years they continued to regard energy devoted to the business as a sign of their caring for their children. When the children had grown and gone, parental illness resurfaced, claiming the time this woman and her husband had anticipated as their retirement bonus. She nursed her husband through a painful terminal illness, determined that she could not run the always-precarious business without him, and, in effect, retired to her home to wait for death.

She speaks wistfully of the painting and drawing she used to do, and she laments that a hard life robbed her of these activities. When asked if she might reclaim them now, when life is not quite so demanding, she replies, "Oh, but I couldn't. It's been years." This woman subordinated her own creativity to somewhat ambivalent efforts at procreativity, and she raised three children whom she now describes as "very dutiful people." They send greeting cards on appropriate holidays, and they send formal announcements of such events as a son's promotion at work and a grandchild's birth or religious confirmation. In response, perhaps, to their limited contact with her, perhaps to her old ambivalence about putting aside her personal interests in favor of attending to the family's needs, this woman gets less vicarious satisfaction than many subjects do, from the milestones of the next generations. During the tempestuous family years, working so hard at a business that never really came alive, she used to long for the opportunity to draw. She tended to think, "If I could make just one picture, I would know I could still produce something good, something beautiful." Somehow, she never found that opportunity. And now she feels that it is too late.

One couple is an instructive exception to the usual pattern, in which procreativity has dominated the lifelong sense of caring. For these people, productivity has always been paramount. Since their teenage marriage, they have operated a successful family ranch in the Sierra foothills. Unlike many other occupations, ranching (California ranching is what is often referred to as farming in other regions of the country) consistently calls for creativity and nurturance, as well as industriousness and competence. Everyday responsibilities include the care of living plants and animals. Over the decades, these people have raised generations of cows and chickens and have tended each year's crop of fruits and nuts —from bud, to harvest, to dormancy care. In addition, the business of the ranch has required its own kind of care, to survive the financial exigencies that result from changes in economic and meteorological conditions.

This couple love their ranch, and they have given it all of the work, energy, and care it has demanded. Their children, too, have been involved in it from their earliest years. A consequence of this familywide, passionate devotion to the ranch, however, is that even when the children were quite small, neither parent had much time to devote to their nurturing. Most of their early daytime child care was provided by grandparents. Once they were old enough, they joined their parents in caring for the ranch. Arrangements have now been made and new acreage acquired, so that all of the children have moved into positions of senior management and responsibility. They will be able to run the ranch on their own when (or if) their parents choose to withdraw from it completely, and the ranch will be able to support their separate families.

It is not that these people have neglected to parent their children. It is, rather, that they have done so largely through mutual involvement in the ranch. It has often seemed, not that the ranch exists as a means of caring for the family, as does the wholesale business of the family discussed above, but that the family exists as a means of caring for the ranch. Today this couple express some regret for the hard work that left them too little time with the children when they were younger. Still, their very real concern for the children's well-being is even today inextricably bound up in their concern for the ranch.

Most of our subjects are eager to talk about current relations with their children—a major realm in which elders are able to reface the interplay between generativity and stagnation. They struggle to balance their ongoing, lifelong concern and feelings of responsibility for their children's well-being with the recognition that as middle-aged adults with children (and often grandchildren) of their own, these "children" deserve to have their independence respected. Central to this struggle is the giving of advice, often perceived as the last vestige of active parenting. Concern prompts the aged to advise. Respect prompts them to refrain from advising.

A few parents seem quite comfortable with the mutual giving, receiving, and ignoring of advice. One mother explains, "I tell my children what's on my mind and vice versa. We can always ignore it." She says she has always been open with her children: "Love and thoughtfulness have always characterized my family relations. We certainly don't say everything that comes into our heads. But we have always been open with opinions and advice, based on love and consideration, and there is no reason that should change. Of course, we respect each other's right to make our own decisions." For her, it seems that the *giving* of advice, regardless of its content, represents parental and filial caring—the expression of which is appreciated in both generations, as it always has been.

Many people try to refrain from giving their adult children any kind of advice, either out of consideration for the children's feelings or out of respect for the next generation's responsibility for their own lives. One extremely energetic, autonomous woman explains, "My daughter and I are buddies. We don't have to rely on each other. We just enjoy each other. Until something comes up and I'm the mother and she's the daughter. That's when I have to keep my mouth shut. She's that way with her own children, too." For this informant, "something coming up" refers to any situation in which she thinks her daughter is making some kind of preventable, potentially damaging mistake. Such situations apparently call forth in her a longtime parental desire to care by guiding and protecting. At the same time, she feels that the stage when it was appropriate for her to prevent her daughter's mistakes has long since passed. This daughter has survived to middle age despite a congenital, life-threatening medical condition. From the beginning, the parents flouted mainstream medical advice in refusing to let this condition turn their child's life into that of an invalid. Throughout her parenthood, then, this subject has integrated generative caring with a profound belief in and respect for individual autonomy and self-reliance. She continues to do so. It is not that in her old age she no longer cares. Rather, it is that she feels that the demonstrations of this caring must change with the changing stages of the life cycle.

For some of the parents in our study, refraining from giving their children advice has origins that are more pragmatic than philosophical. Whereas the making of suggestions and imposing of restrictions may be effective ways to guide young people, these parents have learned that these same kinds of guidance often have undesirable effects on relations with adult children. One woman notes, "I'd like to give the children advice, but I keep my mouth shut because it's so easy to be misunderstood." Another expands on a similar theme: "I control the impulse to give my children advice. I'm careful not to criticize or offer advice, because they never follow it anyway. They resent my intrusion, and they get angry, and they don't even hear what it is that I'm saying. And then, of course, there is a period of bad feeling, and somebody has to apologize. I think that is too bad, because there are many times my advice could have saved them grief and money. But if they won't listen, there's no point in' talking." Each of these reasons for holding back represents a form of learning, on the part of the parent, about how effectively to demonstrate concern for middle-aged children.

The giving of advice is not a one-way practice, but, instead, a mutual expression of caring, between generations. Our subjects wrestle with the tension between feelings of caring and those of helplessness about receiving advice as well as giving it. On one hand, they want to be able to count on the children, to know that they care enough to be relied upon. On the other hand, they feel a self-reliant reluctance to accept advice or assistance from anyone. One mother's observation exemplifies this tension: "You know they make me so mad when they remind me what the doctor says I can and can't eat! If I want to eat a piece of cake and suffer the consequences, that's my business. Still, I know they care, and I'd rather be mad at their meddling than wonder if they even knew about my diabetes." This woman has always tempered her strong will with the good judgment that tells her, today, that her children's dietary reminders do not really threaten her essential autonomy. She strives to accept their sometimes irritating advice with a philosophical appreciation that validates their sense of generativity while involving her in a dimension of old age's grand-generativity. These efforts are all part of her reintegrating a productive sense of intergenerational concern with an opposing tendency toward self-absorption.

Related to the intergenerational exchange of advice is the exchange of assistance. Sociological data suggest that throughout the life cycle, and almost regardless of family socioeconomic status, assistance flows both "down" from older generations to younger ones and "up" from younger to older. Particularly in the middle class, parents continue to provide considerable financial assistance to middle-aged children, even into old age.* Indeed, several of our subjects speak proudly of giving various kinds of financial support to their children's families. Some pay for long-distance telephoning and visiting, or finance family celebrations. Some use occasions when gifts are appropriate to provide necessities like automobile tires, a new roof, or annual college tuition assistance. Virtually all say that they give money to their children and families and that they enjoy making such gifts. Reciprocally, many parents describe receiving some form of financial assistance from their children. In contrast to their ambivalence toward the children's advice, it is with matter-of-fact gratitude that these people accept such major gifts as a car to replace one that was destroyed in an accident and that they receive such gestures of financial support as the payment of moving expenses or assistance with living costs in a partial-care facility. Although they may consider advice largely intrusive, most of our subjects and, by report, their children seem to regard these kinds of financial assistance as appropriate expressions of ongoing affection and concern between generations.

---

*L. E. Troll, S. J. Miller, and R. C. Atchley, *Families in Later Life* (Belmont, Calif.: Wadsworth, 1979).

Along with the financial, many other forms of assistance are comfortably exchanged between our aged subjects and their middle-aged children. Most elders speak with proud satisfaction of the children's general helpfulness. They point to help in such specific areas as transportation, moving, and entertaining, apparently viewing such assistance as an indication of the love and esteem in which they are held. In the reciprocal direction, our informants describe the support they provide to their children as an appropriate expression of later-life caring. They are glad to be able to help. They are even gladder that their family relationships are such that their help is welcome. This sincere satisfaction, like the philosophical appreciation expressed by the diabetic woman discussed above, serves to enhance the children's sense of caring responsibility, in turn strengthening the elders' sense of grand-generativity.

We have noted throughout this section that aged parents' relations with grown children are an important opportunity for demonstrating care in old age and for reviewing and reconciling the caring expressed in earlier life. As part of the generational cycle, our subjects, like other parents, became grandparents as their children matured and became parents themselves. This later-life experience of grandparenthood provides them an additional opportunity to integrate feelings of responsible nurturance with those of less productive self-concern. Research indicates that grandparenthood offers many individuals a "second chance" at generativity. That is, it presents the possibility of caring for the newest generation more robustly, and less ambivalently than they did for their own young children, in their years of active parenthood.*

Of those subjects who are documented as having had diffi-

---

*H. Q. Kivnick, *The Meaning of Grandparenthood* (Ann Arbor, Mich.: UMI Research Press, 1982).

culty parenting, one, in particular, describes taking full advantage of this opportunity: "I have always been perfectly willing to be a babysitter and what have you. I have enjoyed my grandchildren tremendously, from their very earliest moments." This woman was overinvolved in every aspect of her own children's lives, and tension and frustration often permeated her household. Her children were all extraordinarily bright, and she took her parental responsibilities to include the expectation of excellence from them, in a wide variety of often-competing behaviors and activities. In contrast, she describes relationships with her grandchildren as warm, relaxed, and mutually respectful and satisfying—quite unlike those she was able to have with her own children at corresponding periods in their lives. She does not impose her own expectations of excellence. She is able to appreciate the accomplishments that are important to them. In this woman, grandparenthood somehow elicits or permits a concerned, respectful nurturance of which she seemed almost incapable earlier in her life, with the children for whose lives she was responsible. From relationships with her grandchildren she is learning to show her children a kind of supportive concern she has never before been able to demonstrate. For the first time, she is able to hear of their problems and to convey to them, in a manner they can appreciate, her feelings of concern, respect, empathy, supportiveness, and confidence. Not only has she finally been able to participate in critically important dimensions of the psychosocial experience of generativity, through her grandchildren. She also finds herself renewing, and actually repairing, her ongoing relationships with her own, grown children.

With grandchildren, elders may participate in any number of ways in guiding and maintaining this newest generation. All of these enhance the sense of being caring and being

valued as family elders.* But, as grandparents, elders can
contribute to their grandchildren's guidance and maintenance without being *responsible for* them. As grandparents,
they can love, care for, and be helpful to the grandchildren
—all without bearing the responsibility inherent in parental
generativity. This freedom from middle age's responsibility
for maintaining and perpetuating the world is central to the
grand-generativity that characterizes old-age caring. And
this very freedom is something many elders relish about
being grandparents. One observes, "With grandparenthood
you don't have the worry of twenty-four-hour responsibility.
You have plenty of time to play with them, and you can take
things more calmly."

Grandparenting enables elders to reintegrate a wide variety of other dimensions of generativity. In taking the grandchildren for a weekend while the parents go off by themselves, a grandfather is caring both for his grandchildren and
for his children. In loving and admiring the grandchildren,
he is validating his children's generativity—the product, of
course, of his own generativity. For some, it is easier to brag
about their grandchildren than about their children; it seems
less immodest to burst with pride about the grandchildren
than about the children. The distance of this next generation
often allows those of our aged informants who had difficulty
with parenthood, or who simply found it hard to acknowledge generative success, to experience in the grandchildren
the feelings of pride that they could not let themselves experience in their children. In seeing her own blue eyes in a
granddaughter and in recognizing her grandmother's smile
and sense of humor, a grandmother experiences the continu-

---

*H. Q. Kivnick, "Grandparenthood: An Overview of Meaning and Mental
Health," *Gerontologist* 22 (1982): 59–66.

ity of five generations—a continuity that would not exist without her own generative contribution.

For a few of our subjects, grandparenthood has involved long periods of surrogate parenting. One widowed woman was called on to move in with her newly divorced son and care for her infant grandson while her son consolidated his professional and emotional life. This woman had very much enjoyed the daily activities of motherhood, and she had little reluctance about resuming them temporarily. She stayed for six years. In retrospect, she talks of this experience both warmly and sadly. She was sad for her son's divorce—sad, too, that he was unable to function adequately as a father. But she was grateful for the generational bond that enabled him to ask for her help and her to provide it. She came to appreciate the chance to perform, again, the activities she had found so gratifying as a mother, and the unique opportunity to become as close to her grandson as she is now. She recalls, "I was his mom. He called me 'Mom.' I took him to nursery school with a bunch of kids. I PTA-ed all over again —in my late sixties, this was." She goes on to explain that in this capacity she also found herself serving as a kind of adviser to the young mothers of her grandson's classmates: "We would have coffee together, and I guess it's easier for some people to talk to someone who isn't part of their family." Looking back, she feels that her assistance served a necessary function in her family's development. She also expresses relief that this kind of assistance is no longer required.

Some elders demonstrate a deep concern for the impact, positive or negative, they feel they have on the grandchildren. With sensitivity and self-discipline, they modify their own behavior in view of its potential effects on the grandchildren. A sad, desperate woman of eighty-nine says that she

refrains from taking her own life because of how the grandchildren might react. They love and admire her, and she is
a significant figure in their lives. She is afraid they might not
understand her suicide, and rather than risk losing their
respect or dangerously upsetting them, she continues to endure the pain her current life entails. This woman has outlived both her age-mates and her good health. In her daily
life she finds nothing to distract her from endless rumination
about what she should have done differently. She feels that
she cannot now participate in activities that might begin to
bring into balance what she views as the sins of the past. Her
decision not to terminate her life demonstrates a profound
caring for the next generations. She has not discussed this
topic with them, so they will never know of the active caring
that underlies what must look, to them, like her rather passive longevity.

A final hope for generative confirmation resides in the way
various individuals hope to be remembered by the grandchildren, after death. "I'd like them to remember me as a kind
and loving grandfather. A good man, and one who thought
a great deal of them." "I'd like them to think of me as a
fountain of wisdom." "I want the grandchildren to say they
had fun with me." It is almost as if these subjects feel that
confirmation received now, while they are still alive, is less
definitive than confirmation provided after death—as if the
affirmation they receive in the present is less permanent than
the one they hope the grandchildren will provide into the
indefinite future that will exist after death.

Although relationships with children and grandchildren
form the major domain in which the elders in our study find
themselves bringing into balance lifelong feelings of
generativity and stagnation, other relationships, too, call for
the integration of essential care in old age. A number of our

subjects have been involved in caring for seriously disabled relatives, sometimes nursing them through long terminal illnesses. For the past four years a man, now ninety-two years old, and his wife have provided a home for his wife's invalid, eighty-eight-year-old sister. They have supported this woman financially since she was incapacitated several years ago. Now she is completely bedridden, almost completely paralyzed, and apparently unable to be left unattended. For the past two years, this man's wife has slept in the downstairs sickroom. He shakes his head and says, "It's ruined my sex life, but I don't think she did this on purpose. You have to be philosophical about these things." Caring for her takes all of the time and energy our subject and his wife have to give. They are, quite literally, devoting their lives to her care.

This man represents an additional exception to the pattern discussed earlier, that procreativity represents the dominant expression of generativity in middle adulthood. As a young man, he cared deeply about his profession of pharmacy. Long before he was committed to caring for a wife and children, he was committed to his profession and to upholding its highest traditions. He took quite seriously his responsibility for the health of the community. Although he worked long hours at the same kinds of tasks that occupied other pharmacists and storekeepers, the nature of his involvement with his profession always went far beyond viewing it as a series of duties whose completion meant a meal ticket for himself and his family. He was always concerned about the well-being of the profession itself, from its daily activities to its ultimate survival. When "the old pharmacy died, after the war," this man, through no fault but that of societal progress, lost an essential focus of his generativity. Today he looks back on the old-style pharmacy almost as on a deceased loved one. He speaks of it wistfully and with longing.

This subject's comfortable feelings of nurturance toward his profession stand in contrast to prospective life-historical material that suggests he always had difficulty in expressing his care for his children directly. He spent little time at home, and one interpersonal tension or another always seemed to interfere with moments of intimate caring. His own childhood had been marked by his father's abandonment during his infancy, and his mother's death before he reached school age. He was housed by various relatives until, in his very early teens, he left town to make his way across the country. Perhaps the absence of parental or family generativity in his own childhood contributed to his awkwardness with the generativity of his own parenthood.

Today, in very old age, his current involvement in generative caring focuses on individual people somewhat more than in earlier years. He is able to appreciate concerned attention when it is forthcoming from his children, though he feels that he has little to offer them in return. Always philosophical, he addresses his recurrent twinges of stagnation in relation to them, saying, "You give what you can where you can. I always gave them everything I could. Now I have nothing for them. But now they can give to me a little bit, and so they do. It's that simple." Wearier than any of our other subjects, this man seems to have come to terms with his life so that he is ready to die. However, caretaking responsibility for his sister-in-law keeps him alive. Despite obliquely expressed resentment at the way her illness has interfered with his marriage and even with his dying, he observes, "The only thing that keeps me alive is my obligation to the family. . . . [Otherwise] I am willing to die any time. . . . [But] I can't think about leaving now, when this lady depends on me."

Several of our informants care for siblings or cousins who

can no longer be maintained outside institutions. One woman spends every afternoon with her demented older brother, who lives in a nearby convalescent home. She explains, "He would like to live with me, but that is just not possible. My children warned me never to try to care for him at home. He was alone, and he wanted to live with me. He was also incontinent and senile most of the time. I thought the children were awfully cruel, but because I know they really do care about my well-being, I tolerated feeling guilty for a few days and thought about it more carefully. You know, I decided they were right. But I feel so bad. He has no children, so I am IT. And when I am there, he doesn't recognize me. I'm not much good to him just sitting in his room, so while I am there, I wheel people from their rooms and pass out trays. It's so hard to see him go mentally, and not to be able to help."

Generativity has been the major psychosocial strength of this woman's adult life. Until her children were grown, her life revolved around raising them and providing wifely care for her husband. Of all our subjects, this is the one who stands out as speaking with wistful pleasure of such distant child-rearing roles as room mother, scout den mother, and PTA president. She enthusiastically details her children's school projects and special events. She lovingly recalls their favorite outfits, describing the lump that used to swell in her throat as she watched them grow out of each one. When the children left home, she went to work for the Red Cross.

Perhaps because of the conviction with which she has always cared for her family, she felt intolerably self-centered, even in considering refusing to care for her brother as he wished. Perhaps because of the grace that has also always attended her caring, she experienced less ambivalence about receiving advice from the children than other people might have. Characteristically, she is now caring for her brother in a way that maximizes generativity in all family members. She has taken the children's advice in a way that lets them feel that they have cared well for her. She is providing her brother with all the care she can give—in a way that does not leave her feeling bitter, depleted, or unable to care further. In addition, she attends to her brother in a way that lets her care for other lonely convalescent-home residents as well.

Many older people engage in a more mutual exchange of assistance with siblings and cousins. They rely on one another in times of illness, tacitly assuming that such a reliance will be temporary and that it will be reciprocated. In the loneliness imposed by children's distance and by the longevity through which they have outlived their spouses and close friends, they turn to one another for companionship, for reminiscence, and for a good laugh. Each is for the others "someone you know will always care."

Other informants engage in a different kind of reciprocal caring, with people in younger generations. For the past ten years, one woman has housed Asian students for the International House at a local college. By now she has what she regards as a large international family of grandchildren. Initially, she felt primarily that she was in a position to offer a service to these lonely foreigners. Her children were gone, and even with a student or two she still had room for visiting grandchildren. She was somewhat surprised at the warmth and closeness of the relationships she found herself developing with these strangers. Far from simply providing a room, she was providing a home and a family. To her surprise, they were providing her a family in return. She came to enjoy the bustle they and their friends created in the kitchen. She liked stocking the refrigerator with soda and beer. She valued this renewed connection with college life. She loved hearing stories of their home countries. She was touched by their concern for her—by how they would look for things around the house that needed fixing or improving; would insist on accompanying her if she wanted to go out at night; would escort her to campus events they thought would be of interest. As with her grandchildren, with these students this woman is able to enjoy caring and being cared for, free of the parental responsibilities and the years of personal history that may complicate generativity between parents and children.

Many elders demonstrate concern in less intensive ways. One man checks on an irascible neighbor from a distance, looking each day to make sure her shades are raised, her garbage taken out, her garden watered, and so on. Several individuals are part of church- or neighborhood-based telephone networks, through which people phone one another several times a week. In one community, a group of elders have organized a van to take them to the senior center. If one of their number is missing without notice, someone will check up immediately, and each member of the group will provide whatever assistance is within his or her capacity. A woman who is active and healthy delivers "meals on wheels." A woman who is neither active nor healthy crochets shawls and afghans for hospital patients. These aged individuals are no longer responsible for the maintenance of the world as a whole. Nonetheless, they are very much involved in the daily maintenance of one another.

In addition to the specific interpersonal expressions discussed thus far, our informants also show general, communal attitudes toward care. As they review their pasts, they identify lifelong beliefs according to which they have always tried to live—beliefs that reflect an enduring, underlying concern for community, for country, and for all of humankind. We recognize political involvement as an expression of this kind of communal concern. Several of our subjects demonstrate such involvement in their old age. Some describe themselves as "religious" voters. Some contribute money. Some write letters. Some recall earlier-life activity in party politics or nonpartisan voting efforts. Proud of what they worked for in younger years, they reinvolve themselves today. One declares, "I keep a batch of postcards, and when I get too mad I write. Some of these things are so vicious and destructive!" To another, a lack of interest or abstention from participation in the political process is unthinkable. "Your ears always prick up [at an election], and be sure to vote. That is *necessary.*" These people very clearly articulate a diversity of ideas about the impact of various political movements on the well-being of the economy, the morality of children, and the survival of humanity. Although most of them are no longer in a position to exert major individual influence on the course of events, they still view themselves as responsible members of society. For all of them, political participation is an expression of concern for the country and for the world at large. As elders, they are no longer responsible for maintaining the world, but as long as they are alive they will be responsible for a caring participation in it.

A final component of reviewing past caring in old age has to do with considering the role of the generative experience in the individual's overall philosophy of life, that is, with recognizing the extent to which his or her worldview incorporates a broad sense of integral concern for the well-being of the world and its people. One man who describes this kind of broad concern throughout his life is the pharmacist discussed earlier. He recalls that one of the things he liked most about his work was the opportunity to help others. He explains, "I like to help people. I had my own store. I did much paramedic work. I was in a poor neighborhood, and people came to me instead of a doctor, and I helped them. I liked that feeling." As he struggles to integrate a final sense of care, this feeling of community concern helps bring into balance the shortcomings he has never been able to overlook.

Another man continues to wrestle with a lifelong conflict between "loving your brother and making a living." For him, as for many other men, caring and nurturing have primarily involved making a living for his family. However more overtly than many other people, this man also voices concern for the individuals with whom daily life brought him into contact. Unfortunately, he seems to have experienced the very sense of caring that motivated him to work in the first place as being directly incompatible with the attitudes and behaviors necessary to succeed at working. He made his living as a salesman. As he reviews his career, he laments that although he always tried to be considerate of his clients and to give them a fair deal, they did not always reciprocate. Similarly, he tried to respect the territories of other salesmen, and similarly they did not reciprocate. Although he always made a living, he never made either the fortune or the shining accomplishment that he dreamed of. He has always interpreted this failure primarily as a difficulty in balancing concern for himself with concern for colleagues, clients, and competitors. Unable to treat these others badly, he always subordinated concern for himself. This man is still unable to reconcile this tension. He feels that by behaving well toward his colleagues, he in effect cared badly for himself and his family. He struggles with his sense of personal failure and tries in vain to derive comparable satisfaction from having lived out the honorable belief that humankind survives on the basis of our decency and kindness toward one another.

Apart from the roles that nurturance and self-concern

have actually played in these people's lives, each of our informants holds, in later life, a more general view of the role these capacities should play in the world. "I think conservation, [caring for the earth,] is our duty. After all, it's our world while we're living in it." "If I had the strength, I'd get the head of every country together and lecture them, 'Don't you feel ashamed [of your selfish destruction]?' " "It all boils down to learning to get along with people. Along the line you learn how to understand and see the other fellow's point of view." "I feel we are put on earth to take care of each other if we can, and I believe in that." "The secret is to do things for other people." These worldviews all represent the formulations of individuals who have passed from active responsibility for the maintenance of the world. Each one is based on a lifetime of caring and failing to care, evaluated in the face of the knowledge that there is no longer either the time or the power to effect that caring on anything but a small, personal scale. Still, the aged have struggled to put these feelings into words, and they try, in the time that remains, to put them into action as well.

Our subjects are all concerned that today's children receive the guidance essential to their becoming adults in whose hands the world will be safe. Their ideas are surprisingly consistent about how they, as grand-generative adults, must contribute to this guidance. "If you want your child or grandchild to trust what you say, he has to see you all along as trustworthy—as living the way you say he should live. If you do that all along, why, he'll know he can trust you, and that makes you feel darned good." They are convinced that children do not grow into responsible adults as a result of casual advice and classroom lessons. Responsible adults mature from children who live in trustworthy relationships with responsible adults. Children absorb their standards from their elders, in all generations. As the oldest elders in today's society, these people feel that it is their grand-generative responsibility to be trustworthy in their demonstration of the highest human standards.

One last feeling shared by a number of our informants is captured in the comment "I wish I could be young and know what I know now." In particular, people focus on breaches of generativity in the service of self that they wish they had been wise enough to avoid. "You make fool mistakes sometimes, and hurt people when you don't intend to." As they review the influence they have had on people over the years, the aged often recognize injuries they inflicted as a by-product of self-directed goals that, at the time, seemed to overshadow everything else. For many people, the importance of these other goals has long since diminished, in the face of a final reconsideration of the value of lifelong relationships. Their having harmed others in the service of self-interest can no longer be overlooked or justified, as perhaps it could in earlier years. Experiencing painful regret for past offenses, the aged still have the opportunity to demonstrate real caring in the present. It is precisely this process of reconciling the past today in order to live better tomorrow that remains the essence of living with the tensions and challenges of a lifetime.

3. Intimacy and Isolation: Love

Throughout the life cycle, a balance between the capacity for intimacy and the need for some isolation enables the individual to engage with others whom he or she can love and be loved by, with true mutuality. Like the young adult, the elder must reconcile a sense of closeness with the experience of being alone, consolidating once more the capacity for love.

However, in old age the individual faces these issues in the context of relationships that have endured for many decades and of those that are more recent. A sense of love at the end of life must involve a coming to terms with love, expressed and not expressed, over the course of the whole life cycle. That is, in reviewing the sharing and the separateness of earlier years, the elder seeks to keep alive the capacity for love.

Maintaining a sense of loving mutuality in old age is often difficult and painful, as the elder may be forced to confront isolation imposed by the death of a lifelong partner and of longtime friends. In addition, at least some of the children and grandchildren are likely to live at distances that inhibit an intergenerational intimacy based on daily interaction. Thus, it is from a position of often unaccustomed and unwelcome aloneness that the elder must reassimilate the strengths and weaknesses of earlier loving. It is from this same position that he or she meets, in marriage and in other kinds of closeness, those new partners who will share in the mutuality of a renewed capacity for love.

Relationships with people of all ages must give way to new patterns and balances. Inevitable physiological deterioration may make it difficult for old people to negotiate geographical distances or to read one another's handwritten letters. Friends whose intimacy has been based on a sharing of activities may suddenly find themselves unable to enjoy window-shopping or vacationing in the mountains, for example. It may often seem much easier to think with fond longing of friends who are deceased than to expend whatever kinds of effort are necessary to have contact with those who are simply some distance away. Old age's many experiences of isolation challenge the individual to develop and maintain relationships of mutuality with people in all generations.

Our informants include long-married couples, individuals who are widowed and divorced, and ones who are now remarried. (Throughout this chapter we shall use the word *widow* as a generic term, to refer to a man or a woman whose marital partner has died.) Regardless of their current marital status, however, they fondly recall the courtship experiences of their teens and twenties—experiences that marked the beginning of long-term marriages in which they have experienced the intimacy that has dominated their adult lives. For some, very specific memories seem to evoke an immediate, sensual reinvolvement in their earliest adulthood commitments to intimacy. One woman met her husband through his family, and she says, eyes twinkling, "I was crazy about him. We went out together for three months, but he never touched me. Finally I told him, 'Something better happen tonight or else.' I wouldn't explain any more. So he kissed me that night, and he kissed me until the day he died." This woman has now been widowed for many years. She has filled her life with children and grandchildren, and with friends and activities. Because of her lively sense of humor and essential good-heartedness, she is regarded as a welcome companion. But for her no current companion can replace her husband. The love she shares with these others cannot replace the love she shared with him. Perhaps her telling anecdotes about her life together with him continues to evoke in her that particular, special love that she has not shared with anyone since he died.

In the past few years, this woman has become nearly blind and increasingly deaf. Having lost one leg to a diabetes-related disease, she is confined to a wheelchair. Hugs and touches of affection are increasingly important, as they convey several critical messages. Most obviously, they tell her that she is loved, and they allow her to express her love in return. In addition, they supplement the dubiously reliable information provided by her eyes, in letting her know that she is not alone in a room. Finally, this kind of touching conveys, quite physically, the message that although she is old and although she is ill, she is still part of the world of living people, where individuals reach out to one another in body as well as in spirit. Sadly, for this woman as for many similarly disabled elders, fragility tends to keep at bay the spontaneous, affectionate physical contact that is so much a part of old loving. It is primarily with grandchildren that she, like many others, is able to enjoy the loving reassurance of physical contact. Reminiscing about the sensuality of early love enables her to view with life-span perspective the unwelcome extent to which she now remains largely apart. Perhaps, in eliciting the feelings of an earlier time, it also helps fill this current void.

As the sexual quality of long-intimate relationships undergoes age-related changes, and as now-unmarried individuals live in often unchosen celibacy, reminiscing allows elders to reintegrate qualities of earlier-life tenderness, affection, and sexuality. However shyly or awkwardly, many of our subjects describe having chosen their partners on the basis of a measure of sexual attraction. A few people speak openly about early feelings of love and fondness. An extremely conservative man of few words blushes as he recalls that after high school he and his girlfriend (later to become his wife) attended different colleges but "kept on liking each other pretty good." Another man chuckles as he explains, "I met my wife at one of them kissing parties." For these individuals, as for many others, the recalling of earlier sensuality seems to serve as a source of happiness, as it brings to life intimate experience that has been missed for many years.

A few of our informants stand out for having chosen partners quite explicitly for reasons that were practical and social rather than romantic. A man reports that he deliberately married someone who was different from his other girl-friends: "I wanted a good, dependable person who didn't wear rouge or jazz around. Someone whose standards I respected." According to the historical material, one woman seemed proud to marry without either fondness or erotic attachment. After playing the campus heartbreaker for several years, she finally chose a husband for "sensible reasons. He was fairminded and serious about life and money." When this woman was a child, her family was poor and her parents were divorced. Her mother expended great energy vilifying her ex-husband and warning her daughter about the dangers of men and the sexual behavior into which they forced women. Our informant saw her father on infrequent occasions, which she describes as idyllic. From these reunions, she would return home to her mother's barrage. Shortly after she graduated from high school, her mother was permanently institutionalized as psychotic.

At university our informant seems, paradoxically, both to have acted out the role against which her mother had warned her so bitterly and to have acted upon her mother's advice. On the one hand, she is said to have flirted and teased young men unmercifully, taking full advantage of her beauty and her allure. On the other hand, when she finally decided to marry, she chose a partner to whom, historical data indicate, she felt little sexual or romantic attraction—a man from whom she would be able to maintain a measure of isolation. Historical data also indicate that although our informant had anticipated a workable marriage based on sensibleness and fairmindedness, her relationship with her husband soon became permanently distant and cold. Furthermore, historical data include speculations that this distant coldness served our informant as an essential defense against unconscious feelings of fear of and distaste for the husband who was, after all, a man.

In the old age of today, after many years of widowhood, this woman describes her marriage as having been marked by sweetness and devotion. She laughingly recalls her husband's having confided to her that for months before they were formally introduced he would make his morning deliveries on foot so that he could be near her as she walked to her first class. Every morning he would lean on the fence as she passed by, and he would hum "Here Comes Fiona McClaren in Her Bonny Blue Bonnet." More seriously, she continues to recall that she was touched by his devoted admiration and that she felt she would "follow him to the ends of the earth" to reciprocate the happiness he had given her.

This woman's current recollections of her courtship and her marriage differ sharply from her own earlier descriptions and from those of the Guidance Study staff, provided decades ago. This discrepancy suggests that her current reminiscences are serving a valuable psychosocial function in her very old age. In the face of today's loneliness, her recasting of earlier closeness with her husband provides a reassuring kind of company. Family history data suggest that, at the very least, the rudimentary sense of loving intimacy that this woman was able to develop in childhood was riddled with mistrust and isolation. It may be that throughout adulthood her very involvement in the intimacy of a marriage engendered such fright that it sparked the antagonistic feelings and behaviors noted in our historical records. Now, at a distance from the interpersonal intimacy she seems to have found so frightening, she is perhaps better able to attend to feelings of love and closeness that have remained lifelong silent partners to the antagonism she has always expressed. It may also be that, after a lifetime of overt bitterness and isolation, this woman feels she has little time left in which to express a sense of intimacy. Regardless of its relation to documented life history, this expression would seem to be another function served by her particularly picturesque reminiscing about loving courtship and marriage.

Most of the people in our study recall, or at least describe, marriages of lifelong mutual affection, supportiveness, understanding, companionship, and ever-increasing appreciation. A thoughtful man, married in his teens and comfortable today after decades of grappling with poverty and setbacks, notes with real tenderness, "The fondness we had for each other has always eased all other pains." Other informants cite numerous aspects of consistent mutuality and gratification in their long married lives: "We have always shared all our activities and made all decisions together." "We enjoy our own company." "We tried hard to please each other." "We grew closer over time." "We always enjoyed each other so darned much." "We have a better understanding as we get older as a family." "I need him for some things and he needs me. We're complementary." "We were always happy being together and doing things together." All of these recollections are integral to the fondness, devotion, and passion of love in old age.

We find quite striking the consistency and uniformity of these descriptions of marital intimacy, particularly in view of various suggestions, in the files of such informants as the woman discussed at length above, of earlier-life marital difficulties and dissatisfactions. Such discrepancies between today's descriptions and those given forty years ago seem to indicate an important psychological process. They suggest that for some elders, after decades in which the balance between intimacy and isolation was often precarious, integrating a sense of love across the whole life cycle may involve the reevaluating and recasting of earlier experiences to such an extent that these experiences become unrecognizable to the outsider.

Even those of our informants for whom, according to the historical data, difficulties and separateness seemed to outweigh intimate mutuality for decades—even they are reluctant to mention marital difficulties of any sort, past or present, in their conversations with us. On the whole, they prefer to report gratifying marriages of affection and complementarity. The cases of two individuals are particularly illustrative. A woman, a rather recent widow whom, in earlier life, the Guidance Study had advised against the divorce she repeatedly threatened, now describes her marriage as having been "devoted from the very beginning. We were sweethearts to the day he died." For this woman it seems that, throughout the period of child rearing, marriage meant gratifying intimacy in chaotic imbalance with frustrating isolation. This imbalance lessened when the children left home, and for more than the last twenty years of their life together, she and her husband shared an intimacy that was perhaps especially gratifying in its contrast to the unhappiness of the preceding decades. This woman is both pleased with and proud of the mutual devotion of the latter half of her marriage. In her old age, this immediately preceding period clearly dominates her sense of marital intimacy, and it is the one she most wants to remember.

Historical records indicate that throughout her thirties and forties, a second woman reported to the Guidance Study that she had nothing in common with her husband, that they quarreled incessantly, that he was offering little either to her or to their three sons, that she was responsible for him as for an additional child, and that she wanted very much to be out of what she experienced as an oppressive and unrewarding marriage. Today she asserts, "The fact that we think so much alike is one of the strongest ties that has held us together. We have always done everything together. Always helped one another. For sixty-one years." Today, indeed, this couple do seem to do everything together. In a manner often character-istic of people who have known each other very well, for a long, long time, they participate in a gentle, playful teasing, interspersed with matter-of-fact observations about each other's strengths and idiosyncrasies. They figure in almost every sentence of each other's conversation, and they are clearly and inextricably part of each other's lives. The *fact* of this old-age intimacy has certainly transcended the painful marital differences of forty years ago. Still, the disparity between these two views of this marriage remains striking. Perhaps this woman would feel disloyal at mentioning short-comings perceived earlier in the partner to whom she has been so close for so long. Or perhaps years of mutual devo-tion have colored her memories, so that she remembers the early decades of marriage as a time not of argument with each other but, instead, of mutual struggle against the out-side world.

Many of the women in our study came of age in an era of Victorian prudishness that frequently led to ignorance about sexuality. One exclaims, "Can you imagine, six older broth-ers and I didn't even know where babies come from until a month before I was married!" Another recalls ruefully, "I didn't know anything about sex until I was grown and almost married. When I found out I was just sick." Typical of partners in Victorian marriages, many of our subjects seem to have experienced difficult marital adjustments and serious early sexual problems, often characterized by frigidity in women and resigned good humor in men. For most couples,

sincere affection and good-natured patience often made possible marriages that weathered their stormy beginnings and
proved, ultimately, to be mutually satisfying and enduring.
As they seek to reintegrate qualities of fondness, affection,
and sexuality into a lifelong sense of love, the elders in our
study are able to pass over short-lived early difficulties and
to focus, instead, on a long lifetime of marital satisfaction.

Only a very few of our aged informants are explicitly
critical of or disappointed in their spouses or their lifelong
marriages. One woman, now widowed, looks back on her
husband as having been incapable of affection. She recalls, "I
looked to my children for intimacy." This woman does not
speak of her feelings toward her husband during the long
years of their marriage. Historical data indicate that in addition to being incapable of affection he was also unable to earn
a living, leaving to his wife the responsibility of supporting
the family. She met this responsibility and blossomed with it.
However, while she developed certain dimensions of
generativity and industriousness to a greater extent than she
might have if her family and work situations had been more
traditional, she developed dimensions of intimacy to a lesser
extent than most women in more-traditional circumstances.
Particularly since her husband's death, this woman has developed a valuable mutuality in relations with her children.
Today she looks back with resigned acceptance on the absence of closeness with her husband, and she quickly moves
on to consider the more immediate, more gratifying intimacy
she has been able to share with the children. Somehow, she
has been able to balance the isolation in her marital past with
an overall sense of intimacy that exists into the present.

In contrast, the following man cannot put behind him the
sense of isolation he felt in his marriage. Divorced for approximately twenty years, he complains that his wife felt

superior to him from the very beginning: "I often wonder why I married that woman. And to think that I stayed with her for thirty-two years!" This man has been single since his divorce, and his bitterness against his ex-wife still pervades his converation. He blames her for turning the children against him. Although she died several years ago, it continues to rankle that she remarried shortly after leaving him, while he has remained alone. In comparison with the woman discussed immediately above, this man does not seem to have maximized other psychosocial strengths to compensate for the enduring lack of intimacy in his marriage. Neither has he found subsequent intimacy with children or friends. Thus, in old age he looks back on a marriage that failed more than two decades ago, as his primary experience in an intimate relationship. From that temporally distant marriage, feelings of bitter isolation persist with a degree of affect usually associated with events of the present. It is as if he has not been able to relegate his ex-wife or his failed marriage to the past, and so they, and the feelings they engender, remain very much a part of his present.

Among the very few elders who acknowledge disharmony in their present-day relationships are a long-married couple whose current life painfully illustrates several issues that may arise as deteriorating aged partners seek to reintegrate the lifelong themes of intimacy and isolation. This couple present a rosy view of their history together. Theirs seems to have been a rather traditional, highly complementary marriage. On a severely restricted budget, the wife showed enormous energy and ingenuity in raising five children, nurturing their intellectual and artistic talents, and maintaining an interesting and visually attractive home. The husband worked long, hard hours to provide the family's income. Both parents enjoyed their particular family-related tasks.

With respect to the world outside the home, the wife remained perpetually in the background. She facilitated and applauded her husband's achievements. She laughed at his jokes. He always relied on and appreciated her support.

Now the husband observes, "We've been a good balance to each other in the past. But there's not a good balance now." The wife's arthritis forced this couple to move to a bland, ordinary apartment, away from the lovely home into which they had put so much effort, and in which they had planned to live out their days. Her condition has continued to deteriorate, forcing a more recent move into a two-room unit in a facility that serves meals and provides medical and therapeutic care. She dozes off in the middle of conversations, meals, and movies.

Instead of being well cared for by a clever, energetic, appreciative partner for whom he could enjoy striving to excel, the husband is now required to provide care for an often unappreciative invalid. Yet, as hard as he may try, he knows that he cannot provide all of the care she needs. He must arrange for her to receive supplementary professional assistance. He resents being forced to learn the kinds of domestic activities that have never been part of his repertoire. He resents the loss of his cheering section at a time when his own confidence requires boosting. He is angry at her abandoning him with so little notice. He sadly misses his companion of many decades, and he is truly concerned about her deteriorating condition. Searching for other sources of mutuality, he has developed an active friendship network within their building, and he often flees his apartment for companionship.

The wife is resentful of his impatience with her, and she becomes increasingly determined to rely on him for everything. She will not accept assistance from workers who are paid to provide such services as bathing or physical therapy;

she will accept assistance only from her husband. After years of running a household, she is frustrated and embarrassed at being helpless. She is frightened and furious at the perception that when, for the first time in their life together, she has had to be dependent on her husband, he does not reciprocate her years of devotion himself, but, instead, passes the buck by enlisting assistance. Afraid of being without him, she ties him to her with a very short rope. She asserts that she has no interest in being friends with any of the people in the building, but when her husband is visiting with a neighbor, she will phone, insist that he come fetch her, and then somehow be unable to remain in the neighbor's home for more than a few minutes.

This couple represents a poignant extreme in the kinds of adjustments old age and its deteriorations can force long-term partners to make in their expectations of and behaviors toward one another. These people's long-established, complementary patterns of intimacy are no longer effective, and thus far they have been unable to adapt to their perpetually changing circumstances. Each of them feels wronged, isolated, and abandoned. Each feels so angry and frightened that neither seems able to make the gestures that might strengthen them both—gestures toward meaningful intimacy, toward caring cooperation. After nearly sixty-five years of marriage, their intimate, loving satisfaction now derives almost entirely from their past. And this past they describe in terms so mutually consistent, so rigidly unchanging, that the description takes on the quality of a mantra. Perhaps the strength of this consensual, frequently reevoked image of appropriate intimacy will somehow either soothe or outweigh the sense of separateness that now threatens to overwhelm each one of them.

Perhaps this couple's old-age situation will stabilize in

such a way that they will be able to accommodate, to establish a new, workable balance between current intimacy and current individual isolation. Whatever progress they are able to make for the future, today's present difficulties will be part of the past on which they will look back in ten years, as they seek to integrate mutuality and separation across their old age.

Even couples whose physical health does not precipitate such sudden, severe alterations in lifelong patterns must adapt to changes in daily routine, imposed by diminished energy, by professinal retirement, and by new interests and activities. They must adapt to changes in individual trust, autonomy, initiative, industriousness, and identity—in themselves and in each other. And with such adaptation must come the establishment of a new equilibrium between feeling close and feeling alone.

The wife of a new retiree observes, "We get on each other's nerves a little bit. We're not used to being together all the time." This couple face the challenge of developing satisfying patterns of individual independence in a context of physical proximity and emotional closeness. The wife can no longer count on her husband to leave her alone each day and to return home with salary in hand, full of interesting, entertaining stories about his day's adventures as a photojournalist. Throughout most of their marriage, she has devoted her energies to making their home a place where he can relax and "refuel" between workdays. Her vicarious pleasure in the excitement and glamour of his career has long rewarded her for the housework she might otherwise have found boring and repetitive. Now that his career has come to an end, she must look to the past for those rewards on which she has relied, for meeting the household responsibilities that have not terminated along with her husband's employment. She also finds herself with the new responsibility of boosting his confidence. He seems to require frequent reminding that he has not suddenly become incompetent—just retired. Seemingly overnight, the system of rewards and responsibilities on which this couple's intimacy has rested for decades is no longer in its accustomed equilibrium. Establishing a new balance between intimacy and isolation will require both an integration of the past and a reshuffling of the present. And this new balance will itself have to remain flexible enough to respond to the various changes that are likely to confront these people as the years continue to pass.

Among informants who have lost a partner, our interviews usually focused on two primary aspects of widowhood. One of these has to do with the adapting of decades of married living to living a new life, alone. This kind of adaptation by means of behavior represents an important, indirect aspect of coming to terms with feelings like that of the isolation precipitated by widowhood. Such behavior may also be seen as an expression of later-life competence, and it illustrates one of the multifarious interconnections among psychosocial themes in old age. A robust sense of self-confidence and capability can facilitate the reconciling of widowhood's loneliness. Reciprocally, bringing powerful feelings of isolation into scale with lifelong intimacy can enhance the later-life sense of competence.

One practical-minded woman declares, "The crux of widowhood is how much you did for yourself before he died. My sister was a helpless mess." Widowed from a marriage in which she bore lifelong responsibilities for family maintenance and administration, this woman has had relatively little difficulty keeping her finances in order, arranging her own changes in housing, and maintaining an overall sense of order and effectiveness in her day-to-day life. She has not necessarily enjoyed these tasks but is proud that she has been able to accomplish them. Historically critical of those she views as more privileged than herself, she now expresses impatience with peers who were pampered into helplessness over the years. As she reviews a marriage in which she often denigrated her husband's level of achievement, she experiences a new appreciation of the self-reliance this relationship forced her to develop.

Another subject asserts, "You have to get organized and start your whole life all over again." This woman has always believed in doing, rather than in dreaming, as a strategy for solving problems. She has always tried to take advantage of existing resources, refraining from idly envying opportunities that are available to other people. In addition, she has resolutely refused to pay more than passing attention to her inner feelings or those of her family, viewing such behavior as "looking for more trouble, when you ought to be finding a way out of the trouble you are already in." This no-nonsense woman has never liked being alone, and she has always valued close family ties. Within days of her husband's unexpected death, she had made plans to move hundreds of miles, to share an apartment with her sister. Now thoroughly ensconced in her new home, she explains, "You make your life wherever you are. There's so much to do, you just don't have time to mope around, missing those people you don't see any more."

A second major aspect of widowhood concerns coming to terms with the feelings that surround the death of a longtime partner. Closeness and mutuality with their partners have, consciously and unconsciously, been part of every facet of many of these people's sense of themselves. Losing a partner, then, is like losing a part of themselves. One individual mourns, "She was half of me. The family. The house. Even my job and my little projects. I never did anything, but thoughts of her were part of it somewhere. What would she think of a book? Would a joke make her laugh? She is part of everything I look back on. She was part of everything I looked ahead to. Her death was just like a regular sword, and it has to heal in time." Regardless of longtime marital harmony or conflict, these people describe the death of a spouse as a horrible wrenching of an internal world. This same man continues, "We knew she wasn't going to last too long, but when she really died, why, it was just like cutting my world in two." Having lost his partner, this man, like other widows, seeks to come to terms with the intimacy of his marriage, and also with the isolation it involved.

The mourning process seems to provide the opportunity to experience currents of sadness, guilt, passion, resentment, delight, fear, and the many other conflicting emotions that were part of a lifetime of marital love. One man who had come to take his wife's companionship for granted finds himself vividly recalling details of their long life together, every time he looks at the chair in which she used to sit and in which she recently died. A woman speaks of her angry frustration at her husband's leaving her with so little notice or time for preparation, perhaps reflecting other resentments that historical data have documented in this marriage. Expressions of resentment soon give way, however, to memories of the intimate devotion and mutual delight that seem to have predominated in the half century of this couple's love for one another.

Among our informants, widows of long-intimate marriages never really finish with the reexperiencing that is so much a part of mourning. Rather, they seem to reach a point at which these feelings no longer dominate every minute of every day. At this juncture, they find themselves able to begin to build upon the lifelong strength of marital love, in developing new kinds of mutuality with relatives and friends who are still alive. Still, even those individuals who successfully organize their lives in such a way that they spend time with loving friends and family, engage in activities of interest, and participate in programs that provide various kinds of assistance to others—even they often find themselves missing their partners profoundly, after many years of widowhood. They try to be optimistic about this feeling of isolation. A woman explains, "I like to be alone in a way, and I don't really feel lonely. But it is hardest getting along without him because we were so close. I miss his companionship so much." In grappling with this ongoing emptiness, aged widows must continually reconcile the extent to which the lifelong sense of marital intimacy is an inextricable part of old-age identity. These individuals cannot feel like themselves in old age without considering the partners who were part of their lives for so long. In the absence of these partners, a measure of isolation seems to be a necessary dimension of widowhood identity.

Of those widows who have remained alone, most speak quite explicitly about being uninterested in marrying again. A woman laughs and says, "When my friends ask if I don't want a husband I always say, 'Of course! I need three—one to manage the finances, one to maintain the house, and one to keep me company.'" She adds, "When you get old everybody can kiss you, and you're not a threat to anybody." Her humor and perceptive observation hint at the strength of the intimate bond she still has with her husband. Although he is dead, she remains married to him; marriage to someone new would be tantamount to bigamy. This woman does appreciate male company, and she is often grateful to have a man escort her to a nighttime event she would otherwise not attend. She would, quite possibly, be grateful to a man who offered to manage her finances or her household. But although all of these functions are part of the everyday balance of responsibilities making up a marriage, in themselves they concern shared maintenance activities and not the mutuality of marital love. For some women, remarrying may represent a breach of loyalty to their husbands. For others, it may represent an impossible abandonment of a part of themselves. For still others, its challenges may seem to require more energy than they can muster—to face, anew, issues of sexual and emotional intimacy. Although many of these women may wish for assistance in meeting maintenance responsibilities, most seem to view a search for a new marriage partner as all but unthinkable.

Also among the widows in our study are some who are either currently remarried or widowed for the second time. These individuals provide interesting insights into an old-age integration of successive marital intimacy. One man was widowed in his early fifties, when his wife died of cancer. Now in his early nineties, he has been married to his second wife for considerably longer than the twenty-three years he spent with his first. He explains, "I compare the two marriages, but not too much. I never bring up my first wife in conversation. This wife is attentive. She loves me, and I know she does, and I love her. But you can love two people, you know. For a long time, I didn't think about my first wife, and now as I get older I am starting to think more about her." He goes on to speak of his belief that when he dies he will be reunited with his first wife and will spend eternity with her: "I know other people who feel this way, too. One fellow, he really loved his second wife. But when he was dying, it was the first one he called for. No matter how it may seem betweentimes, the first love is the one that lasts forever."

A remarried women feels much the same way about first and second marriages, although her circumstances are quite different. Her first husband died after a long, serious illness, and she says, "I was a widow months before he died, completely, in my mind." They had married young, and she had enthusiastically devoted her life to being the appropriate wife for a man in his constantly rising corporate position. At the time of his death, they had achieved considerable financial and social status. Her second husband is of a different social and economic stratum. They are relatively recently married, and their relationship rests on mutual enjoyment and affection rather than on shared social or professional achievement. She explains, "When I die I know I'll be reunited with my first husband. We belong together. And my dear second husband will be reunited with his first wife. He loved her far too much ever to spend eternity with anyone else."

In the minds of our remarried subjects, marriage in youth and marriage in later life seem to represent two different kinds of intimacy. Marriage in youth appears to imply the fusion of individual identities in mutual intimacy, and these people view this fusion as permanent, regardless of the interventions of death or remarriage. In contrast, marriage in later life seems to represent a commitment to companionship. Although that commitment involves intimacy, sacrifice, compromise, and reciprocity, although it may be expected to last for the rest of life, it nonetheless remains separate from the early, intimate fusion that seems to transcend death and time.

Another indication of the sense that real marital intimacy is not interrupted by death is the acknowledgment by several widows that they have been visited by their departed spouses. They all differentiate these visits from dreams of visits, which they also describe having had. The first person to mention such visits says simply, "My wife still comes to see me. I write it down in this astronomy diary we used to keep together, alongside what stars I see each night." He goes on to explain, "I wasn't asleep. And it wasn't a dream. Her body was real and substantial, and when I held her she was real. And when she left, it wasn't that I just woke up—because I wasn't asleep. She told me good-bye, and she left my arms, and then, as she moved across the room, she slowly began to fade away. I was awake the whole time. It meant so much to me to see her and to hold her those few times." This man recalls having met his wife in a high school game of spin the bottle, and his early sensual involvement with her has clearly endured.

No other subjects volunteered information about such visits, but when explicitly asked, a number of them seemed quite relieved and eager to describe their experiences. One woman recalls, "A few days after my husband passed away, I was awake in the morning and I was crying. And I looked up and I saw him at the foot of the bed, just as plain as anything, just as he often stood after coming in from his early-morning chores. And he said, 'It's all right Mom.' " Another explains, "Sometimes you feel his presence. Not like a ghost appearing, but you know that as long as you don't turn around he'll be there right behind you. You can feel him almost touching you, comfortable and reassuring as always."

Among the individuals who acknowledge having been visited are those who respond to questions along these lines with suddenly tearful exclamations: "I wish he would come to visit me like that!" "I have prayed for so long that he would come to see me. And if other people have come back, then I still have cause for hope." "I wish I had had some visits. O God, how I wish for a visit like that!" These people seem to regard the notion of being visited by a departed spouse as a meaningful part of old age's sense of lifelong intimacy. Whether or not they themselves have received such visits, none of them disregard or disdain these experiences in their peers.

A spouse is not the only person with whom elders have shared meaningful intimacy. Although most of our subjects describe earlier times when family responsibilities took precedence over contact with friends, many now point to friends with whom they have been able to remain close, in one form or another, over many decades. For some people, these friends are coworkers or early mentors. For some, they are members of clubs or activity groups whose regular meetings were part of the weekly schedule, even during child-rearing years. For others, these friends date back to high school or college. Some find that siblings are becoming such friends. To the extent that intimacy includes an element of mutual understanding based on shared experience, each one of these surviving, longtime relationships provides the elder with an intimacy that becomes particularly precious as other forms of closeness and companionship give way to inevitable loss. One woman alludes to the special intimacy that results from shared experience as she describes her current relationship with her ninety-six-year-old sister: "We always tell each other how nice it is that we can laugh about old times, and know exactly what we're laughing about."

Of course, these longtime friendships are a kind of intimate involvement that cannot readily be replaced at the death of one partner. Much like long-term marriages, old friendships may be tied up with a sense of lifelong successes and failures, and with personal development over the years. Much like the loss of a spouse, therefore, the loss of a long-time friend may represent a loss of the intimacy that has persisted for decades. For example, one woman observes,

"My closest friend from college passed away suddenly. We used to do a lot of things together, and I don't do those things any more. We used to talk together in a certain kind of way, and I don't talk in that way, about those kinds of things, any more. I *have* missed her!" Another explains, "My younger sister always brought out certain qualities from my mother in me. I was nicer to her than to anyone else, and it always made me feel so good just to be around her. I don't know if I'll ever feel that good again." As they must in widowhood, elders who lose longtime friends must continue to confront the reality that lifelong intimacy is an integral part of identity in later life and that some measure of empty isolation must be accommodated as a dimension of outliving old friends.

Companionship is an important component of intimacy in the current lives of our informants. However, even this seemingly straightforward yearning for mutuality exists in perpetual tension with forces leading toward isolation. In their marriages and long-term friendships, these people had developed workable balances between these two opposing needs. Now the vicissitudes of aging require them to reevaluate the ways in which they have come to terms with closeness and aloneness. In addition, such a reevaluation often takes place in the context of relationships with new friends—people whom they do not know well and of whose strengths, weaknesses, and special personal needs they are not sure. Many long for someone to talk to, while recognizing that *"just anyone* isn't necessarily someone [they] could really talk to." For some, it often seems easiest to be alone.

Our subjects report widely divergent patterns of new friendship in their current lives. Some speak with a kind of social disdain, demanding to choose their friends in old age as they did in younger years, on the basis of quality and not simply of proximity and imposed living conditions. Some,

like the following man, long for the kind of friend they seem
unable to find. He sighs, "If I could just find a man or two
to relate and chat with and walk around with. But they are
all busy with their crippled wives." Some philosophically
eschew "getting too chummy with your neighbor," preferring to "do things with friends but keep intimate conversations inside the family." Some make a distinction that increases with age, between friends and acquaintances; they
note in an aloof tone that they are not inclined to make new
friends as rapidly as in earlier years. These expressions of
disdain represent a tendency toward isolation.

Other elders more resiliently find themselves open to involvement with the people and communities at hand, noting,
"Everybody is interesting and has some good quality, if you
bother to look for it." Some individuals observe that they find
themselves feeling quite close to people whom, in younger
days, they might never have chosen to get to know. Others
find themselves participating in informal networks, taking
real responsibility for one another's ongoing well-being.
They check in regularly with each other, providing reliable
contact and sincere concern, and making sure that no one is
in need of something the other network members could provide. Each of these patterns represents a different kind of
balance between old-age intimacy and old-age isolation, serving aged men and women well under some circumstances
and, optimally, giving way to new patterns as these prove
unsatisfactory.

With increasing age, many people find themselves quite
intimately involved with family members of many generations. In some cases, these relationships are not unexpected
outcomes of years of more-distant caring. For these people,
new forms of compatibility and sharing with siblings, children, grandchildren, and nieces and nephews seem to arise,

almost of necessity, as older expressions of love become impossible. For example, some elders report that the death of a grown child has occasioned a new closeness with those children who remain. A special new intimacy among survivors seems to emerge when the deceased individual was important to all of them, and this intimacy may be a form of mourning and a new bond between members of all generations.

Widows often emerge from the loss of a spouse in newly intimate relationships with children, siblings, and other relatives and age-mates. One woman recalls that her children were very attentive to her at the time of her husband's death, and she observes that since then "they have taken very good care of [her], in ways they didn't used to." They are concerned that her car be maintained in problem-free running condition. They support her rejecting of new obligations that she feels she should take on but that would, realistically, be far too burdensome for her to discharge at this time. This woman has always been close to her children, has always been concerned for their welfare, and has always provided assistance at critical points in their lives. But it is only since the death of her husband that she has begun to accept from her children the kind of concerned caring that she has always offered to them. The individual ways in which this mother and her children experienced isolation at the death of her husband, their father, and the ways in which they have empathized with one another's isolation have all brought a new mutuality to their closeness.

Many elders devote more and more energy to appreciating and assisting the children who have stepped in to try to mitigate losses imposed by death, disease, and distance. One woman has lived with her daughter's family since immediately after she was widowed. Before this move, she and her husband had gone to great lengths not to play favorites among their many children. Now, however, she asserts, "Doing things for my daughter and her children is my total livelihood right now. They are so wonderful to me. They let me cook for them, read to them, tell stories with them. I don't think they could do anything I might want to criticize." While this woman's husband was alive, her paramount concern was with his happiness. He was the source of her delight, and she tried to delight him in return. Now that he is gone, she demonstrates a similar attitude toward the daughter and family with whom she lives. The members of this family are now her major source of caring and vitality. She appreciates them more than she can express, and she "would give them the world if it was [hers]."

4. IDENTITY AND IDENTITY CONFUSION: FIDELITY

Old age's reconciling of the tension between identity and identity confusion reinvolves the individual in the psychosocial process that dominated adolescence. The elder faces the task of bringing identity and a sense of identity diffusion into balance by seeking to make sense of the self that has lived through many decades, that lives in the present, and that will continue to live in the indeterminate future. In reviewing a lifetime of beliefs faithfully held, and of personal characteristics that have endured without benefit of conscious commitment, the aged individual is in a unique position to reevaluate experience with the perspective of time. In comparing early hopes and dreams with life actually lived, he or she struggles to come to terms with the realities of personal capacities in an individualized context of uncontrollable life circumstances. Balancing a lifelong sense of continuity with that of discontinuity or diffusion, the elder also faces a last opportunity to make, and to act on, commitments that best reflect the "I" in the totality of life—what we may call existential identity.

The older person's generational identity differs from earlier-life perceptions of the self in the generational cycle. For perhaps the first time, the elder is a member of the omega generation, the oldest living generation in his or her family. There are no other living elders to whom to look for guidance through the next stage. Members of the omega generation must be guided by ideological heroes and by their own wisdom and memories, as they themselves serve as guides for the generations that follow. The sense of identity in old age rests not only on recollection and evaluation of the personal past but also on members of younger generations and on their representation of the generational future. In the final stage of the life cycle, a sense of self is grounded not only in the personal choices and actions of a lifetime but also in the generations that will survive the elder and that will remember him or her into the future.

From adolescence, the individual's sense of identity derives from personal commitments to beliefs and attitudes, and to activities and relationships that reflect these beliefs. During adulthood, the individual struggles to balance a faithfulness to some commitments with an inevitable confusion and abandonment of others, all the while living a life that, in turn, both represents and reflects an underlying sense of self. In old age, however, physiological deterioration, interpersonal losses, and a variety of societal circumstances all tend to confine the individual's life. Activities that have long been expressions of personal identity may be restricted. Relationships on whose interpersonal reflection the elder has long relied in order to experience an enduring sense of self may be eliminated or unrecognizably altered. In the face of a diminishing number of familiar representations and reflections, our subjects struggle to reconcile their sense of who they have been during their long lives with a newer, ever-changing sense of who they may yet come to be in old age.

An old woman who has long identified with being classically beautiful must somehow accept the image her mirror now reflects—perhaps faded, perhaps intensified—without retroactively invalidating the physical beauty that was hers until recently. A ninety-year-old who broke her nose running for a bus when she forgot that she "wasn't young any more" must somehow temper her spirited sense of energy with behavioral respect for her own physical fragility.

A lifelong PTA and community group organizer who, with increasing frequency, finds herself almost too tired to make a telephone call clings to her identity as a networker as a way of "keeping old age licked." She explains, "If you force yourself to keep going, then you keep feeling like yourself. The minute you give up, though, you're gone." Her observation suggests that the characteristic fear of old-age disability and overall incapacitation plays an important role in the later-life integration of identity with identity confusion. That is, our aging subjects struggle to continue to feel like themselves at a time when they must also accept the fact that they are no longer capable of enjoying those longtime appearances and activities from which they have come to derive a sense of themselves.

Many people emphasize lifelong continuity. They point to characteristics that highlight a sense of self, as if to remind themselves who they are, what they believe, and how they must continue to look at life. For example, one woman asserts, "I pride myself on being cheerful and sensible and keeping busy. I am a happy soul." This woman left school to enter a marriage in which she and her husband "were always happy together": "I could make him laugh, and everything was swell for us." Enthusiastic as a full-time housewife and mother, she served as president of the PTA, leader of church youth groups, and director of regional scouting activities. When the children left home, she joined political clubs and women's social organizations. Immediately after her husband's death, she suffered a heart attack. However, in keeping with her sense of herself as "a rebounder," she recovered quickly and began to travel. She was reluctant to be sick any longer than absolutely necessary and was eager to see new places. In coping with her husband's death, she found it important to continue to be interested in the world and its people, to continue to meet new people with whom she could enjoy laughing.

More recently, osteoporosis has led to her falling and breaking numerous vertebrae. Using characteristic good sense, she curtailed her travels in favor of the vicarious exploration inherent in reading. Most recently, deteriorating eyesight has made reading difficult. Today this woman is very active in her church. She participates in a regular prayer group and is part of a network of church people she describes as her family. With each setback, she has relied on a continuous, underlying sense of herself as a woman who lives in the world in a particularly active, involved way. As important people and activities have disappeared from her life, she has substituted new people and activities in such a way that she continues to demonstrate the same qualities of interpersonal cheerfulness and and sensible busyness that have characterized her for the past seventy or eighty years.

In a variety of ways, the individual involves other people in the process of integrating a sense of identity with feelings of confusion. One aspect of developing a sense of self involves the making of commitments to others with whom one can identify, that is, with whom one shares fidelity to a set of values. Over the course of life, the individual seeks to balance the image he or she sees reflected from these others with the more personal images seen from within. In old age, these external images are particularly important, as they represent the ways the individual will be remembered after death. That is, they represent those elements of identity that are sure to have a future, after the individual has died. For example, one woman declares, "I'd like to be remembered for having humor." In recent years, however, this woman seems dour. She is much more likely to leave people bristling than to fill them with mirth. She was married to an inveterate jokester, and for more than fifty years she enjoyed being entertained by him. From the moment they met, she appreciated this humorous quality in him and valued the reciprocal qualities it elicited in her. She knows that without him this important part of her identity remains hidden. But she has certainly not abandoned it. In singling out humor as the quality for which she would like to be remembered, she is identifying it as an important part of herself. She is also conveying the extent to which her own enduring identity, the image that will remain alive after her death, is intertwined with her husband and their marriage.

One man recognizes and regrets his lifelong shortcomings. In old age he observes, "I'm not a whiz at personal success through other people's eyes, but I enjoy the things I do. If people want to listen to what I have to say, that's fine, and if not, I guess that's okay, too. I believe in what I'm doing, and I'm certainly not hurting anyone." This man never made a particularly good living. Because of illness and limited skills, he was out of work far more often than many of his peers. His family suffered chronic financial uncertainty, and throughout middle age he was confronted with images, both reflected and projected, of himself as an incompetent and a failure. In more recent years, however, new criteria have emerged for his evaluating of failure and success.

When the children were grown and this man could retire, he and his wife left the city in which he had never felt at home, to take up residence in a cabin in the High Sierra. Life was harsh under these rustic conditions. This couple were directly responsible for keeping themselves fed, sheltered, and warm. No longer did success depend on satisfactorily completing a boss's assignments. Instead, it was a function of meeting the direct challenges of nature and of working together with the other people in the area. This man and his wife blossomed in their new surroundings. "We may not do things the way anyone else would, but we do them our way and it seems to work out all right," he explains. Away from externally imposed failure, he has found a new satisfaction in talking with other people, in listening to what they think and in learning from their ideas. Particularly since his wife's death, he has begun to consider the identity that he hopes will survive his own death in the form of memories in the hearts of friends and family. He says simply, "I'd like to be remembered as 'He listened to what I said.' "

For some of our informants, old-age identity as a unique, accomplished, successful person seems to rest on a patronizing attitude toward other old people. One man has long cherished a sense of individuality as one who possesses great, still-untapped talents that set him apart from all others. Proud of his inventive interpersonal style, he speaks with both resentment and a kind of pity about "those old folks around here, who have nothing on their own, and they imitate my way of doing everything." A lifelong, driving intellectual scoffs at the lowly interests of the other old residents in her building, explaining that she would never try to talk with them, because they could offer nothing to interest her.

These two informants have, throughout life, identified themselves on the basis of favorable comparison with their peers—in their own eyes and in the eyes of others. For both of them, identifying with success has implied being more successful than others; being intelligent has implied being more intelligent than others. This kind of comparative identity has always involved a measure of disdain, of repudiation of various "other" identities, and in later life it continues to do so. However, in old age it acquires additional dimensions. Societal circumstances and stereotypes concur in suggesting that with increasing age the individual is likely to experience diminished competence and success, according to the evaluative criteria used in earlier stages of the life cycle. These two subjects are particularly sensitive to general societal criteria, for they have always used them as a source of self-esteem. Suddenly, they find themselves condemned by their own lifelong standards and relegated to the masses of "others" to whom they have always considered themselves superior. They have great difficulty integrating this element of realistic identity confusion, and in order to maintain faith in the identities they have relied on for so long, they carefully distance themselves from their age-mates.

Social and financial status are important to the lifelong identities of several individuals who characterize themselves in terms of the longstanding privileges they have enjoyed. Some of these people continue to translate privileged opportunity into privileged behavior. In a style and spirit consistent with earlier-life behavior, they continue to take advantage of economic well-being in order to travel, for example, and to treat children and grandchildren to experiences they would otherwise not be able to enjoy. Other subjects, who no longer engage in earlier prerogatives, continue to identify with the *status* of privilege. They may no longer be well enough to travel or energetic enough to entertain, but they derive a proud sense of continuity from recalling and retelling the experiences their money has bought in the past.

For some of our aged subjects, status and identity are bound up in the belongings they have acquired and inherited over the years. The course of authenticating family heirlooms as valuable antiques, for example, can come to represent a kind of personal "credentialing" process. Although a life measured by accomplishments may not be viewed with satisfaction, that same life may acquire a sense of personal status and respect in connection with valuable possessions accumulated. One woman disparaged herself in commenting, "If I wanted to go into the Peace Corps, I wouldn't have one single thing to offer. Terrible. I'm not productive, period." This woman had inherited a number of oil paintings that proved to be quite valuable. During the process of having the paintings authenticated at a major museum, she became acquainted with a number of curators and collectors. She enjoyed their respect as an owner and appreciator of valuable art, and she became friends with one curator, through whom she has developed considerable interest in and knowledge about English and American painting. For perhaps the first time in her life, she feels that she can regard herself as a bona fide expert.

Some elders seem to derive a very different sense of identity from their belongings, using them as concrete reminders of experiences and relationships that are central to the lifelong sense of self. A disabled old man sits in a particular chair and reinvolves himself in the experience of buying that chair, many decades earlier. The young man who bought that chair has long since disappeared, but he comes alive in reminiscence. He reminds this informant of the youthful energy and power that are part of his lifelong identity, even in the weary frailty of old age.

A woman who keeps a basket of rocks and minerals on her reading table reminisces about the mines in which her father worked when she was a young child. The family's life was hard in those days, but its members learned to help each other and to value love and support above fine clothes or fancy food. These are the values according to which this woman has lived the rest of her life. The rocks remind her of where they came from and of how long they have been part of her.

Many people use photographs to evoke the sense of identification that is bound up with particular people. A man hangs on his walls the photographs his wife took on all of their vacations, throughout more than sixty years of marriage. They do not travel any longer, but the experiences they collected together will always be part of each of them. Some elders celebrate their ancestors and their own childhood by adorning their walls with old, formal, photographic portraits. These old photographs remind them of the roots of their identity and, at the end of life, plant them firmly in generational history. Many also celebrate their progeny, displaying snapshots of the children, grandchildren, and great-grandchildren who represent their generational immortality. They rely on photographs as indications that the children's zest and the ancestors' fortitude, as well, were part of their identity long before they began even to think of growing old.

An important dimension of old age's balancing identity with confusion has to do with the elder's capacity to articulate what he or she has believed in, has stood for, over a whole lifetime. Our subjects point to early ideal figures as the source of particular values, placing their own identities in an

historical perspective. Several people identify quite consciously with parents and grandparents. A woman observes,
"We have been able to have a happy home, just like my
parents had." A man notes, "My grandfather was a very fine
man, a fine Christian person." Both of these subjects have
tried to emulate in their lives the qualities they admire in
their forebears, and they are proud to think of themselves as
having carried on with the examples set by these respected
elders.

Other informants hold as role models such family members as an uncle or an older brother. A woman proudly
recounts her oldest brother's story: "He was a self-made
man. He was hardworking and kind. He started out with five
dollars in his pocket, and he built the best store in town.
When someone burned down his store, why, he was able to
make a go of it because the community loved him and
wouldn't let the bosses run his business into the ground."
There is much that this woman admires about her brother:
the optimistic confidence and diligence with which he built
a business from nothing; the kindness, honesty, and dignity
with which he always dealt with customers; the courage with
which he started over after losing everything; the deep love
and respect he earned in his community. When this woman
was a small child, her brother was a source of comfort and
encouragement under difficult circumstances. After he left
home, she consciously tried to emulate the spirit in him that
had been so important to her. Throughout adulthood, she
would think of the success he had made of himself, by living
according to the simple values they had both learned from
their parents. She still regards him as a kind of hero, and her
feelings for him are today very much part of her sense of
herself.

Our informants have, quite naturally, also engaged in the

process of striving to be *unlike* some individuals who presented themselves as potential role models. One man matter-of-factly recalls having patterned himself away from everything embodied by his hated father, saying, "I detested his ways of thinking and behaving, and I tried to develop the opposite. I think I have succeeded." He regards his father as "one of the harshest men" he has ever seen. Strong in will and strong in body, Father was a rancher who sternly disciplined his children and brutalized his wife. He took no pleasure in life. He drove himself hard, deriving no satisfaction from his accomplishments and keeping to himself all feelings except his terrifying rage.

Our informant worked his way through high school and college, largely in order to have a career that would enable him to work at a desk, in a respectable office where people wore suits and spoke to one another in civil tones of voice. More so than any other man in our sample, he actively participated in the daily tasks of running a household and raising young children. He helped his wife with the cooking, cleaning, and shopping. He read the children bedtime stories, cared for them when they were sick, helped them with their homework, and shared in their after-school activities. As he looks back at his life, he is proud of his professional achievement and of his involvement with his family. But he is perhaps proudest of the extent to which he has been unlike his father.

The individuals just discussed illustrate various ways in which elders seek to come to terms with the lives they have lived and the beliefs they have held. In considering success in and satisfaction with their pasts, they find themselves evaluating the effectiveness of the very elements of identity they are trying to reconcile. They all continue to try to live their current lives in terms of the belief systems they have developed over decades. At the same time, however, they are also, often unknowingly, involved in modifying their philosophies of life in order to conform to the lives they have lived. Out of this iterative process of evaluation and modification emerges the personal system of values, beliefs, and characteristics that comes to exemplify each elder's existential identity —that is, what his or her unique existence is coming to mean.

Throughout the life cycle, the individual reviews the tension between identity and identity confusion from successive vantage points, resulting, optimally, in a sturdy sense of fidelity. This developmental, maturational quality of lifelong identity also leads to elders' observations of changes in themselves over time. For example, one woman notes that she has become more compassionate as she has grown older. She has always cared about people, but in earlier life her own identity centered on thinking independently as she struggled to survive from day to day. Money was always in very short suply, and in her efforts to make ends meet for her immediate family, she responded to other people's opinions, behaviors, and circumstances primarily with a quick evaluation of their relevance to her own condition. Sometimes she was critical. Sometimes she was approving or grateful. Always her own family's well-being was the central concern in terms of which outside people or ideas were considered. With the perspective of old age, this woman experiences a diminished necessity for immediate action. Her family is grown, and she herself is secure enough that she is no longer preoccupied, each day, with ensuring tomorrow's survival. For the first time, she is free to translate her lifelong sense of caring into an empathy with people whose conditions are quite different from her own. On the basis of a lifetime of experience and of rather narrowly defined, personalized caring, this aged woman is able to view other people with a new compassion for and understanding of themselves in their own circumstances.

In old age, time for solitary reviewing of the past is essential to reconciling the psychosocial tensions of a lifetime. Some of our subjects say they relish this time alone—time to themselves, in which they can think their own thoughts without distraction. One man developed the style of a loner early on, in order to make the best of a bad social situation. Having long ago grown accustomed to this way of living, he now finds it comfortably familiar and is able to experience pleasure in being alone. Without the need to accommodate to what is, for others, a major social discontinuity, this man is able to enjoy the later-life solitude that is both circumstantially imposed and psychosocially essential. Many of our informants, however, do not enjoy the amount of time they find themselves having to spend on their own. They have lived among people, and it is not by choice that they now find themselves without a social milieu.

Part of the old-age process of reviewing the sense of oneself across the life cycle involves a coming to terms with perceived mistakes, failures, and omissions—with chances missed and opportunities not taken. Now the inescapable winding down of life clearly indicates that there will not be time to return to roads not taken, which may all along have remained part of an underlying sense of identity. Many of our aged informants speak wistfully of aspects of deferred or bypassed roles. They endeavor to integrate, rather than resolutely deny, the mixed feelings that inevitably result from comparing the life actually lived with the life anticipated in youthful fantasy and imagined, over decades, as waiting to be claimed at the next opportunity.

One man is seriously troubled by the fact that he never received the public acclaim that he envisioned in his childhood dreams of becoming an actor or a politician. Even as he struggles to master this disappointment, he is able to experience essential satisfaction regarding aspects of the identity he chose to live out. He reasons, "My goal was to be a storekeeper, and to raise a family, and be healthy, and I did all of those. Have some fun in between, and that is all there is to a life. You don't really need the adulation of a million people, to have your name on the front page of the paper, or things like that." Although throughout the life cycle we may reevaluate choices we have made, our doing so in old age offers what is likely to be a final chance to make changes in roles to be lived in the time remaining as well as a last opportunity to come to terms with roles already lived.

In coming to terms with identity lived, several of our subjects express a kind of life-historical perspective that we regard as unique to the relationship the aged can have with integrity and despair. One woman muses, "I always wanted to teach, and I have recently really wished that I finished school. But at the time I had compensations. Getting married and raising a family. Nothing could have made me happier, and I think that was the right choice for then. But I might be better off now if things had been different then." She continues, "If I had finished school and been a teacher, I would have that sense of accomplishment forever. And I would be able to do so much more, now that I am alone, if I just had that education. I might be a better adviser for the grandchildren, too. At least I wouldn't be so far behind." Now, in old age, this woman is able to consider both the long-run advantages and the long-run disadvantages of early choices, in a way that earlier life simply did not allow. Only at the end of life, after choices have been made and lived, after consequences have been faced in reality rather than merely being anticipated in imagination—only at this point can an individual really know the later-life ramifications of early-life choices. And this woman is wise enough to understand two critical aspects of such a life-historical perspective. First, as a young woman she could not possibly have foreseen life, with the same uniquely accurate perspective she has acquired in old age. Second, the very fact that she is old enough to have this perspective, that is, to have seen consequences that extend over the entire life cycle, means that she no longer has the time to make a wholly different set of choices. Coming to terms with lifelong identity as a pattern of doors opened in good faith and doors left shut in equally good faith involves understanding both of these aspects, and it calls for moving on with integrity, to open or shut those doors that remain to be encountered.

One way in which some elders grapple with past tensions surrounding their own life choices is to take on a measure of a new identity as a fledgling ancestor, a progenitor of the next generations. All of our subjects speak with pride of the professional, financial, and familial achievements of their children and grandchildren. Those individuals who are relatively comfortable with their own identities take self-confirming pleasure in the ways in which their children and grandchildren have followed in their paths. However, even those who are disappointed in themselves are often able to identify with the next generations' success in the very areas in which they themselves have fallen short. In so doing, these disappointed elders are able to expand their views of themselves to include the next generations and their triumphs.

Personal identification with success in the next generations was discussed earlier, as a dimension of reviewing lifelong generativity and stagnation. The fact that this identification also emerges in a discussion of lifelong identity and identity confusion suggests a close connection between these two psychosocial themes as they are reconciled in old age. Although we are considering the themes separately as a gesture at clarity, we must emphasize that reviewing the eight psychosocial themes in old age in no way represents eight independent processes. Rather, the themes represent a set of perpetually intertwined concerns, inseparable by virtue of their lifelong interconnections as the essential motifs of the life cycle. Earlier in this book, we made it clear that at each stage of life, vital involvement in the worlds of people, materials, and ideas is the essential basis both for bringing into balance the psychosocial tension then focal and for reexperiencing and preexperiencing the tensions not currently focal. In old age, as well, themes are intertwined in such a way that involvement in a particular relationship or activity (for example, identification with the succeeding generations' triumphs) may be related to the elder's reconciling more than one psychosocial tension.

A lifelong frustrated musician strongly identifies with the daughter, son, and granddaughter who demonstrate musical and artistic talent. As we discussed with respect to his reintegrating generativity and stagnation, this man has identified himself as a talented and promising musician, for as long as he can remember. However, throughout adulthood, societal and economic circumstances conspired with self-doubt and led him to subordinate serious music to other vocational pursuits. Persistent ambivalence about these choices contributed to another aspect of this man's lifelong identity—as a failed musician. For much of his adulthood, this identity as a failure made it all but impossible for him to take pleasure in the musical accomplishments he did have. Rather than viewing his advertising jingles as an ingenious way both to make a living and to remain at least peripherally involved in the world of music, he viewed them as an ongoing indication of his failure as a serious musician. In addition, while he was always parentally proud of his children's artistic achievements, he was unable to avoid comparing their achievements with his own perceived failures. In the old-age role of patriarch, however, his sense of his own success is dependent upon the accomplishments of those in the next generations. When discussing his family, this man invariably moves quickly to his three musical progeny, empathically describing their frustrations and enthusiastically praising their successes. Although he has not wholly laid to rest his own identity as a failed musician, he finds himself able to take increasing pleasure in a new identity as the source of musical talent and success in his family of procreation. Thus, lifelong identity can in old age take its place in the generational cycle, permitting the satisfactions of vicarious identification to increase in importance, while individual failures begin to pale.

Many elders feel that the values with which they identify and according to which they have lived their lives have now passed from societal dominance. Among our informants, many feel that they have built their lives on the basis of hard work, perseverance, belief in God, and unshakable commitment to family and close friends. These are the values to which they have been faithful since their adolescence. They express dismay that today's dominant ethos seems to regard luck and seizing the moment more highly than setting a goal and working until it has been achieved. They are similarly distressed at what they perceive as society's fascination with anything new and its indifference toward long-term commitment to relationships, religions, or principles that "may not be flashy, but that have kept us all alive when we respected them." Although they do not see their own values reflected in society as a whole, some of our informants are reassured to see them reflected in their own children. One man observes with satisfaction, "My daughter is conservative, careful, and thorough like me. Her house is always clean, and the table always has a fresh cloth, like ours." Rather than dwell on their frustration with the ways in which society has departed from what they believe to be right, people like this man try to focus, instead, on the deep satisfaction they experience at seeing that they have successfully renewed their own beliefs through their children.

Other elders, whose progeny do not reflect the values of earlier generations, find themselves confronting new belief systems, forced either to integrate them or to accept the consequences of identifying with convictions that are regarded as outmoded and irrelevant to today's decisions. For example, one woman who has always eagerly identified herself as a mother and family woman is shocked to hear her newly married niece assert that she will have children only when she and her husband are earning enough to be able to absorb the expenses of a family without changing their lifestyle. On the one hand, our informant violently disapproves of this attitude, regarding it as selfish and shortsighted. Certainly, it challenges the value system with which she has identified for the past seventy years, and she is both angered and threatened by it. On the other hand, this woman has also always demonstrated a fierce, unwavering loyalty to those she loves, and she deeply loves this niece. Her greatest pride is that she has always lived for her family—to make things good for them inside the family, regardless of what their lives may involve in the world outside. Until now, she has had a major influence on the family-related values espoused by the next generations, and she has long relished the role of wise family elder. Suddenly, all of this is called into question, and she finds herself compelled to reevaluate what she believes in, and what she rejects, as an aged member of a family and a society.

Another woman describes her feelings about this kind of situation by explaining, "As an old person, you've had experience, but sometimes it isn't in keeping with present times." In these terms, today's elder must reface issues of identity and identity confusion by seeking to integrate current caring, love, faithfulness, competence, purposefulness, willfulness, and hopefulness in contemporary society with earlier-life values, beliefs, and commitments. This final integration is essential to old age's consolidation of a lifelong sense of oneself.

5. INDUSTRY AND INFERIORITY: COMPETENCE

In old age, the individual continues to renew a sense of competence based on resources from within, on demands from outside, and on opportunities that arise. During its time of ascendancy, this psychosocial theme challenges the school-aged child to balance a tendency toward industriousness and accomplishment with an opposing one toward inferiority and ineptitude. The child struggles to learn facts and to master skills; in so doing, he or she begins to consolidate the strength of competence, deriving both from abilities demonstrated and from feelings experienced. Throughout life, this strength remains grounded in observable behavior as well as in less observable emotions. In later life, it builds on the integration of a lifetime of ability and inability. Particularly in the face of the physiological and sensory deterioration that, in old age, diminishes longtime skills dependent on physical strength, sensory acuity, and fine motor coordination, a lifelong sense of effectiveness is a critical resource. It enables some elders to persevere with integrity, in activities whose performance is no longer as effortless or as flawless as it may once have been. It enables others to experience a sense of later-life capability by reviewing earlier industriousness and inferiority, that is, by recalling earlier involvement in work and, to a lesser extent, in school.

A separation from the work setting may engender a sense of inferiority by removing the individual from many areas in which he or she has participated with competence. However, while retirement deprives the elder of accustomed demands and opportunities for professional accomplishment at work, it may impose its own demands for skillfulness and offer its own opportunities for industriousness. Thus, the aged retiree is challenged to transcend inevitable sources of inferiority. He or she must draw on a lifelong sense of effectiveness in order to become involved with new kinds of learning and activity that build on longtime mastery, and to develop latent interests into newly manifest capabilities.

Changes in the technological, social, and political world may render obsolete those skills and attitudes that earlier formed the basis for a sense of competent involvement in the community. In addition, as the elderly face the increasing imminence of death and the specter of serious disability, for themselves and their age-mates, they confront our ultimate inability to conquer or master this final inevitability. Although we are not able to cure death or eliminate disability, the elder demonstrates a measure of effectiveness simply by acknowledging the imminence of the former and by adapting to the limitations imposed by the latter—and continuing to live with vitality, nonetheless. The people in our study struggle to maximize those longtime capacities that are still available and to find new expressions for the skills, knowledge, and worldly wisdom developed over the course of a lifetime. In addition, they come to value the vicarious experience of deep satisfaction and pride in the achievements of the next generations.

The majority of our subjects, both men and women, have been involved in the world of work, tools, and production. This is the world we recognize as society at large, as that realm of adult life in which, more than any other, industriousness is considered related to success. However, today's old men and women have participated in this realm quite differently. For the men, it has always been the focus of adulthood achievement. For most of the women, the world of remunerated work yielded to one of home-based effectiveness, as the primary domain for the expressing of mastery.

Whether domestic or extradomestic, the world of working involves adults in carrying out responsibilities, struggling to balance feelings of hard work and inferiority, perseverance and inertia, accomplishment and failure, completion and exasperated abandonment. Recalling and reconciling these earlier experiences of working, the aged seek to integrate a sense of lifelong competence on which they will be able to draw in the years that remain.

Before marriage, the women in our study were employed in such fields as housekeeping, playground supervision, fashion merchandising, journalism, schoolteaching, private music teaching, and various forms of clerical and secretarial work. However, all but three suspended such extradomestic industriousness, either to marry or to raise children. These women vary widely in the amount of pride with which they now recall their early work experiences, and the variations reflect differences in individual feelings of mastery, both as they existed in terms of early work and as they have developed in the intervening years. For some of the women, early employment seems to have been a financial necessity from which they were only too glad to be freed by marriage. They were far prouder of their husbands' ability to support them than of the skills for which they themselves had been paid. Others very much valued the stimulation, the responsibility, the remuneration, and the sense of competence involved in working. They left work reluctantly, at the insistence of husband, in-laws, or parents, and they still regret having lost a valuable domain of mastery.

One spirited erstwhile stenographer left northwestern Montana at eighteen and traveled alone across the country to do war-related stenographic work in Washington, D.C. She returned west after the war, and continued to work for several years after her marriage, until the family's car and furniture had been paid for. She left work because she wanted to spend more time raising her children. She recalls, "I was a darned good stenographer. I enjoyed the work, the responsibility, and the fact that I was good at it. Darned good." This woman seems comfortable with her history of serial competencies—first employment, then family, then community politics, then small-time ranching or truck farming. Such a history not only provides her with a sense of generalized industriousness but also demonstrates her ability to master new skills and to adapt with enthusiasm to changing circumstances.

The lifelong capacity for industrious adaptability has been essential to this woman's vitality in establishing her current life as a widow with several chronic medical conditions. Recognizing her physiological limitations, she sold the family's hilltop acreage shortly after her husband died, and moved into the nearby town. She chose a ground-floor apartment with its own patio and small plot of ground so that she could continue to practice the gardening that has always brought her such pleasure. Although her children and grandchildren live far away, she decided to remain in the area in which she had spent most of her adult years, near longtime friends and as part of a community in which she already knew how to live. Shops, transportation and medical facilities, and other services were all familiar to her, and she had no need to grapple with the disorientation often faced by elders who move to unfamiliar communities.

As her physical capacities change, this woman finds herself enjoying an ever-changing sequence of interests—some long dormant, some modified from earlier skills, and some seeming to emerge for the first time in old age. For example, at one time she enjoyed expressing her lifelong expertise at cooking and found satisfaction in developing tasty recipes that conformed to her dietary restrictions. After a while, she decided that this kind of cooking demanded too much energy for the satisfactions it provided, and she turned her industriousness to reading about all the things she would have studied if she had stayed in school. Reading for long periods strained her aging eyes, and most recently she began to write semiautobiographical stories, typing out for grandchildren and for various magazines her stories of farming and mining in the old West.

Several women became involved in some kind of training or employment during the Second World War, and for many this national emergency seems to have provided a welcome opportunity to demonstrate hitherto unexpressed industriousness. Some were preparing to support the family in case their husbands were drafted. Others worked in order to feel that they were making a responsible contribution to the national military effort. Most of them continued in their new jobs for some time after the war was over, apparently deriving satisfaction from accomplishments outside the circumscribed arenas of home and family. One had never been eager to work for money but, once she had started, was surprised to find herself determined to put in enough time to earn a pension. Another discovered that she enjoyed the interpersonal contact and stimulation of what had initially been volunteer labor with the Red Cross. Because of her social skill and administrative competence, she was added to the professional staff of the organization, and she recalls, "That gave me tremendous confidence. It was a feeling that I was doing something worthwhile, and doing it well." Although this woman has long since retired from her job, she continues to be involved in activities she considers worthwhile. For example, she delivers "meals on wheels" and does volunteer work at a nearby nursing home.

Three of the women in our study have been engaged in full-time work outside the home throughout most of adulthood. For all three, as for many of the men, industrious competence in the workplace has been the primary psychosocial scaffolding of their lives. They maximized work performance over home-based effectiveness. Valuing hard work, task completion, and unflagging perseverance above other qualities, they strove to imbue their children with these same values. To some extent, they seem to have used work-related pride and success to compensate for disappointment and to defend against inadequacy experienced in relation to home and family. The following two stories illustrate two very different sets of dynamics associated with this somewhat atypical emphasis.

The first of these lifelong workers is one of the youngest and formally least well educated of our women. Beginning in childhood, she worked hard at home and at earning money outside the home. She asserts, "Mother had very high standards for us," and she acknowledges that she was the child who took on the responsibility of helping Mother raise all the others. She married young and from the outset worked alongside her husband on the commercial ranch that they bought and from which they derived their income. When the children were growing, she bore child-rearing and household responsibilities as well as her share of the ranching labor. She has always regarded work as an enjoyable part of life, "especially work outside the house." In the ranch, she has always been a full partner to her husband. The bookkeeping was her responsibility. She also worked tirelessly, seven days a week, helping with whatever physical tasks needed doing.

This woman performed her work with the capability and industriousness that have always been her major strengths. She has little use for shoddy work or for the shirking of responsibility, and she affirms that she has tried to teach these same values to her children. All of the children have become involved in the family ranch, and most recently its management has been turned over to them. This woman has just turned seventy, and her current sense of herself as a worker rests on her ongoing involvement in helping the children run the ranch, on the splendid health that supports her continuing efforts, and on her pride and pleasure in the children's competence.

A second lifelong working woman was the daughter of two teachers, and she learned quite early in life to value being a good worker. Confused and frightened in childhood by an inconsistent, often angry father, she struggled to weigh the excellent work she did in school against the shame and inferiority of which she was accused at home. This woman married a man who was temperamentally similar to her father but who, unlike him, was never able to earn a living. For most of her married life, therefore, it was her hard work that supported the family. Quite successfully, she has held several responsible, semiadministrative, bookkeeping positions, and she declares with satisfaction, "I never had a job I didn't like; I was very fortunate in my whole working career."

She is exceedingly pleased with her work history. She particularly prides herself on never having failed adequately to discharge the responsibilities with which her bosses entrusted her. After retiring nearly two decades after official retirement age, she took a new job. Only recently, in her late eighties, has she altogether retired from the world of employment. This woman has maximized a primary strength of industry, subordinating capacities for intimacy and care. Her marriage was unsatisfying, and her children were very difficult to raise; she experienced major inadequacy and disappointment in marriage, housekeeping, and child rearing. Competence at work has enabled her to compensate for what she might otherwise have experienced as overwhelming inferiority in other areas of her life. Now that she is no longer employed, she relies heavily on the sense of competence she developed over the past seventy to eighty years. In addition, she is hard at work writing a family history and making plans to have it published. She has involved her children in this project, eliciting their editorial suggestions on her manuscript. Although in earlier adulthood she subordinated family relationships to the responsibilities of working, in old age she seems to be able to use her industriousness as a medium through which to relate to her children with more intimacy and caring than had earlier been expressed between them.

As we have noted, the two women just described were able to maximize the psychosocial strength of competence in the face of frustration and disappointment at meeting the challenges of other adulthood themes. In old age, both can now rely on this lifelong sense of mastery as they review earlier tensions and seek to integrate the themes of later life. In contrast, other women were also frustrated in the home-based tasks of adulthood but were unable either to find or to take advantage of opportunities to maximize other strengths. These individuals have a much shallower reservoir of psychosocial strength on which to draw in reconciling old-age integrity and despair.

One such woman met her husband while working in a clerical position. Their relationship seems to have been bitter and quarrelsome for many years before they were finally divorced, and she feels that from the beginning of their marital difficulties he tried to turn the children against her. Although her husband was perpetually angry with her, he grew even angrier when she left the house for recreation or discussed the possibility of finding a job. In any case, she did not wish to return to clerical work, and she lacked necessary training for the glamorous careers for which she felt real excitement—decorating, designing, and dancing. Now in her early eighties, this woman is bitterly bereft. Alienated from her children, she asserts that they took advantage of her when she had something to give. She does not know whether she or her husband is responsible for their having subsequently rejected her. Quick with indiscriminate admiration for the achievements of others, she has a sense of personal competence that seems to rest primarily on the extent to which she can effectively blame her current poverty and loneliness on lifelong circumstantial pressures rather than on her own feelings of inferiority. She complains, "My closest friends don't think I'm anything. And they can do so much. They entertain beautifully. And they fix everything. I'm not like that." She admires film stars who "started with nothing and have really made something of themselves."

Among the men in our study, a sense of competence in old age seems to be closely related to mastery expressed earlier, in the workplace. These individuals worked in a variety of fields and achieved varying levels of professional and economic success. For many of them, experienced competence and inadequacy seem to have dependeded, throughout life, far more on the kinds of rewards they were receiving than on how well they felt they were doing their jobs. It is as if any particular job and its specific tasks and requirements were subordinate to the overriding concerns of earning a living and of "getting ahead"—of advancing within a company or a field, and of receiving commensurate financial recognition. The following man exemplifies this stance.

He worked hard as a traveling salesman and writer of advertising slogans and jingles, supplementing his salary by buying old houses, repainting and remodeling them, and selling them for a profit. Although he enjoyed writing slogans and remodeling houses and although he knew he did these things quite well, he never enjoyed his job or took a pride in it. He felt himself to be perpetually underpaid, financially insecure, and professionally inadequate. A decade before his retirement, his realistic sense of financial insecurity impelled him to change fields and put in "ten years of dogged effort in a different kind of [sales], to earn the money to pay for our retirement." He violently disliked his new line of work and never felt either honest or competent in what he was doing. Nonetheless, he was meeting financial goals for the first time in his adult life. His pride in the security he earned in his last ten years of employment now supports a new and still-fragile sense of accomplishment. The feelings of inferiority that have plagued him since childhood are balanced, at least to some extent, by a realistic sense of mastery, based on his recent demonstrable success.

Four men describe having had to earn money for their own support ever since childhood. All four of them worked hard and well, putting long hours into careers from which they emerged far better off, financially, than their parents had been. Three of them speak with great pride and satisfaction of what their decades of effort have created—a manufacturing plant, a successful ranch, a high-yielding portfolio of investments. For these men, industriousness has been a driving force, always building on itself and on previous successes. All three espouse an ideology of conscientiousness, effort, ambition, enterprise, discipline, and constancy; they have lived out this ideology, and it has brought them a great sense of satisfaction and success.

The fourth of these early workers is less satisfied with what his efforts have created. Orphaned and seriously injured as a child, he got his first job as a delivery boy for a drugstore. He worked his way across the country, took training in pharmacy, and, after working long hours for a number of different bosses, eventually earned his own store and attained a measure of financial security. This man was no less ambitious, no less hardworking, and no less competent in his profession than the first three. His measure of financial success has been considerably smaller, however, and despite the financial security he now enjoys as a result of his career, disappointment seriously interferes with the pride he would like to feel in nearly seventy years of hard work.

He speaks, somewhat wistfully, of the respect he once received from people in his profession and in the community at large. He was a good druggist in the days in which druggists served as supplementary doctors. He knew he was an important part of his community, and his customers did not let him forget it. He would probably have liked to be able to derive enough satisfaction from the respect he was receiving, and the human contribution he knew he was making, to provide a reasonable counterbalance for the good living he felt he was not earning. But even while they lasted, these dimensions of industriousness never seemed as important to him as the financial rewards, which he always considered inadequate.

This druggist's sense of professional competence suffered the critical midcareer blow of professional obsolescence. He explains, "I made pills and suppositories and tablets and lotions and tinctures and elixirs, and they all went off the market very suddenly and the new lines of goods came in, and all I had to do then was count pills. I missed compounding medicines, because I was good at it. I enjoyed the prescriptions scale and the tablet triturate outfit and the suppository machine." The pharmacist's new role as pill counter did not command the community respect this man had enjoyed by virtue of his earlier activities. Thus, the sudden changes in his field eliminated the professional expertise that supported both his sense of skillfulness and his special, respected status in the community—the two major sources of his sense of competence. What is particularly poignant about this man is not that he lost his major arena of mastery but that he did so long before old age and retirement, at the height of his real skill.

With retirement from salaried employment, most elders lose, or at least undergo major changes in, the areas in which they express and experience primary competence. In addition, they forfeit the sense of accomplishment that often accompanies the bringing home of a regular paycheck. Several men describe dissatisfaction in retirement. A storekeeper who retired at seventy-eight says, "I was happier when I was working. I wouldn't have retired at all except for the holdups." An accountant explains, "I was able to save a lot of businesses from going under during the Depression and the war. I knew what I was doing was worthwhile. I don't have that feeling about what I'm doing at this point." Another retired worker recalls, "I knew how to do things no one else in the agency could do. I was kind of indispensable, and I miss that."

Some of the men in our study retired because, as one noted, "I felt like I deserved to lie around and relax. Take the chance to be lazy." For those who are enjoying retirement, however, the primary satisfaction does not seem to come from open-ended relaxation and permissible laziness. Rather, it seems to derive from new expressions of skillfulness and perseverance—expressions that are possible because these men now find themselves at home with no more pressing demands on their time. Several diligently pursue new or modified hobbies, turning old skills and lifelong industriousness in new directions. Some have used their retirement years to do building and remodeling work on their primary homes, vacation houses, and rental properties. Others have taken to raising exotic plants and to gardening and landscaping for themselves, their families, and community groups and neighbors. One man has restored an old car.

Some have developed new kinds of involvement with the fields from which they are retired. A real estate agent has experimented with personal financial investing, both in real estate and in other areas. This experimentation leaves him financially more secure now than at any other time in his life. The rancher discussed above still helps out in the orchards when needed, but he has begun to do the kind of small-scale, exploratory agricultural research for which he has never before had time.

The old age that comes upon all retirees sooner or later confronts many with new, often unwelcome tasks. After a lifetime of partnership, caring for a seriously disabled spouse can be both frightening and burdensome. Particularly for men, this may be the first time in their lives that they have had to provide consistent nurturance and maintain a functioning household. Learning these new, specific skills may certainly be expected to threaten inferiority. One man has overcome early feelings of inadequacy, and he now experiences some satisfaction at caring for his deteriorating wife in a way that enables her to remain in their home. More important than his initial unfamiliarity with shopping and cleaning, however, has been his unfamiliarity with a situation that he can neither master nor reasonably blame himself for failing to conquer. In his work life, he either succeeded or sought to understand how he should have behaved differently in order to succeed. By contrast, he has been able to do nothing to arrest his aging wife's deterioration. She can hardly walk or dress herself. Pain medication leaves her perpetually drowsy and unresponsive. She is withering away before his eyes, and he has been able to do nothing to stop, or even to retard, the process. Although he is pleased that he has been able to keep her out of a nursing home, that satisfaction often seems small in comparison with his knowledge that she is dying and that he is absolutely incompetent to do more than watch.

All of these postretirement involvements have in common the fact that, at least to some extent, they are motivated internally, practiced on the basis of self-discipline, and evaluated on the basis of intrinsically experienced adequacy. Retirement has freed most of the men from their overriding life's work of earning a living, and several of them are for the first time able to evaluate how well they can use their capacities in personally chosen activities. In contrast to the job-related paradigm of accomplishment that is experienced primarily in terms of external rewards received, these men are now deriving satisfaction from the experience of competence as integral to activity itself. The psychosocial demands of later life and their differences from those of youth and middle age seem to allow some old men to enjoy this dimension of industriousness, which they were simply unable to regard as meaningful in earlier life.

Some men have not been able either to continue to pursue lifelong interests in work activities or to find new involvements. For these individuals, meaningful accomplishment in old age is missing. For them, therefore, the current old-age experience of industriousness, skillfulness, and perseverance is, at best, precarious in a way that threatens their lifelong sense of competence. One man clings to increasingly incoherent stories of business successes in earlier life. Since his retirement, he has done little but sit in a wheelchair, inside his mansion, recalling the glories of building and managing a profitable manufacturing firm. The presence of servants has always made it unnecessary for him to be industrious in caring for himself or his home. His interests have never extended very far beyond the walls of his factory, and since he stopped working there, he has not been able to find a new domain in which to demonstrate competence. He answers all questions, regardless of their content, by talking of what is on his mind. And what is on his mind is the myriad emblems of success that he accrued before retiring from his job and that he insistently recalls in an effort to shore up his diminishing sense of mastery.

Another man begins to denigrate earlier achievements in the light of a perceived present inadequacy. In his late eighties, he no longer provides an income for his wife and himself. He is no longer strong or agile, can no longer make small repairs on his home. He now lacks the endurance to complete a game of chess. These current sources of inferiority outweigh the sense of industriousness that he developed over decades of successful employment. Although historical information indicates that he was capable in his field, he now speaks cynically not only of being inadequate today but of having been inadequate all along as well. Rather than drawing strength from the accomplishments of younger years, he seems today to be giving way to a retroactive identification with the inadequacies of his old age, and to be relinquishing the sense of competence developed over a lifetime.

The women's issues around changing competencies in retirement are quite different from those experienced by the men. Those women who were married when their husband retired began their own retirement at the same time. Some terminated long-term employment. Others retired by curtailing such volunteer activities as book reviewing, political work, and fund-raising and such recreational activities as social clubs, sports and games leagues, and lecture series. Similarly to the way men viewed earning a living as the lifelong task for which competence was critical, these women seem to have viewed the managing of household and family as their primary lifelong domain for the exercise of skillfulness and expertise. When that home-based domain could be easily managed, as it often can after children have left home, there was time for volunteer jobs and for recreation. However, whereas retirement freed the men from their lifelong focus of industriousness, it simply changed, and often intensified, the quality of that focus for the married women. That is, a husband's retirement returned him full-time to his home, thus changing the nature of the householding to which his wife had become accustomed over the preceding years, and necessitating major rearrangements of her time and energies.

Some women describe being quite satisfied to spend time and share activities with their husbands. They seem to regard the providing of companionship and the accomplishment of housework as demonstrations of effective competence in later life, and they express little regret over abandoned arenas for other kinds of mastery. One woman explains, "I retired when my husband retired, and I stopped going to most lectures and meetings and things. I did miss the people at work, but my place was with him. For so many years he was so busy at work that it was just a pleasure to be able to be together, and for me to make our life pleasant and comfortable."

Some women, however, feel uncomfortably lazy and stagnant in this kind of retirement arrangement. For them, outside activities had become an important realm of involvement in industriousness, and a valuable source of satisfaction. Increased commitment to householding and companionship with one's husband does not seem to compensate for the loss of these outside satisfactions. One woman relates, "My husband says retirement is like the measles. There is nothing you can do about it." This is a woman who had abandoned her early professional aspirations at the insistence of her husband and family, and who seems, over the years, to have accepted the designation of more dependent, less accomplished partner. Extradomestic involvements had gradually become an important domain in which she could be competent, away from family scrutiny. It may well be that, for her, the home represents a situation in which she has never been able to feel truly capable. If so, returning to it full-time may signify a return to an earlier, unhappier sense of inadequacy.

For all of those elders who live independently, maintaining the home retains some association with a sense of industriousness. Particularly among the men who live alone, the need to keep themselves fed and clothed, the house in order, and the bills paid may catalyze the development of an entirely new set of skills. Some widowed women regard the home as the primary arena for the expression of competent functioning, as it has always been. They continue to take pride in their cooking, cleaning, and entertaining. They may redecorate a room, have the yard landscaped, or care for the gardens of their children or neighbors. When they relocate, they put great effort into setting up the new apartment and are quite proud of their efforts. More so than others, these women are likely to experience extreme inadequacy if temporary illness or injury or long-term disability makes it impossible for them to continue to perform these tasks effectively.

For one woman, in particular, old-age householding represents a new challenge for developing competence. This woman dropped out of college for reasons that apparently included both physical illness and a lack of confidence in her ability to complete her major on schedule. According to prospective data, after marriage she was never very successful in the home. It is not that her primary activities were elsewhere. They were not. But her tendency toward nervous overinvolvement in her husband's and children's lives seriously impaired her effectiveness in household-related activities. Her current enthusiastic involvement in redecorating her home represents a critical reintegration of the tension between industry and inferiority—a tension whose earlier-life balance was, for her, unsatisfactory. As we noted earlier, different developmental stages place different kinds of psychosocial demands on the individual. Under the youthful demands of schooling and the earlier-adulthood demands of raising a family, this woman was unable to reconcile a sense of mastery with her overriding feelings of inadequacy. Now, under the less interpersonal demands of later-life widowhood, she finds herself able to demonstrate industriousness and to experience a measure of accomplishment. In so doing, she is taking advantage of a valuable opportunity old age offers to many elders, that is, the opportunity of one more chance to make things right.

As many men regard retirement as freedom from the need to earn a living, so some women regard later life as liberation from the lifelong link between housekeeping and female adequacy. Several explain, with some satisfaction, that they have always disliked housecleaning, that new energy limits are forcing them to choose activities carefully, and that other things are now obviously more important than a tidy or orderly home. Rather than regretting that they have lost the capacity to maintain their homes at earlier standards, these women seem almost relieved to have an excuse to develop new and different interests. One, as was noted earlier, is quite diligently involved in educating herself: "I'm reading all the classics I've never had time for before." Another puts considerable effort into writing short stories and having them published. A third is having a long autobiography published in book form. A fourth has become an avid folk dancer, practicing for hours each day, watching experts, and performing in exhibitions around the Bay Area. For all of these women, self-declared freedom from one domain of industriousness has provided an opportunity to take advantage of new, hitherto unexplored domains.

Competence in old age is inevitably subject to comparison with competence at earlier ages. Since all of our informants suffer from some degree of physical deterioration and decline in strength, all must come to terms with being less energetic, less proficient, and less effective in executing various physical and cognitive skills than they were in their younger years. Some people reconcile this decline by revising their criteria for adequate accomplishment. Rather than expecting to be able to put a once-commonplace sixteen hours into yard work, for example, they may identify specific tasks whose completion provides a sense of mastery. One man says, "Now I feel satisfied when I accomplish whatever it is that I set out to do. Like rake the leaves out back. It doesn't have to be the back and the front, and the pruning and the dormant spraying. I feel satisfied when I set out to rake the back, and when I've done it."

Several people have modified lifelong hobbies, responding with industriousness and ingenuity to age-related limitations. For example, a longtime painter no longer has the space, the patience, or the physical tolerance to stretch canvases, mix oil-based colors, or work with a palette. In recent years, she has taken up cartooning, which she can do with a pencil or a pen and ink; she now devotes considerable time to drawing cartoons that spoof the retired elderly.

Some individuals attempt to deny their diminished capability altogether. One woman, for example, describes keeping house for her only son, who, she explains, was injured and permanently incapacitated in an automobile accident. Delicate and frail-looking, this subject opened the door into a small living room whose windows couldn't seem to let in enough light to relieve the perpetual darkness. She seated herself with great difficulty, and her shaking hands could not lift a teacup to her lips without spilling its contents down the front of her wrinkled silk dress. During the course of the interview, a young man she introduced as her son bustled through the front door, bags of groceries in each arm. She asked what he was planning to cook for dinner and what time she could expect the meal to be ready. He answered her questions, brought us fresh cups of tea, and then disappeared into the kitchen. Through a closed door came sounds of creaky old cabinets being opened to receive new purchases and banged shut again, and the rest of the interview was accompanied by the muffled chugging and whooshing of a washing machine and dryer.

The decline in lifelong skillfulness poses a major challenge to the sense of mastery in old age. Unless the individual can find some way to meet this challenge, like those discussed above, he or she may be overwhelmed by feelings of inferiority and generalized despair. Earlier in this chapter, we identified effective participation in the world of work, tools, and production as the means by which individuals maintain involvement in society at large—in the communal world of adulthood. This participation remains an ongoing source of the lifelong strength of competence. When the physiological disabilities and constricting societal opportunities of old age make it difficult for the elderly to maintain a realistic effectiveness, what is at stake is nothing less fundamental than their sense of participation in the world of adulthood. A depressed, seriously disabled, wheelchair-bound woman observes sadly, "There isn't much I can do. I can't clean. I can't cook. And that was my life, cooking and cleaning—ever since I stopped being a little girl. There isn't anything left of *you* when you're old."

Aside from individual losses of specific areas of capability, the social, political, and technological changes occurring over the course of our informants' long lifetimes seriously alter the kinds of day-to-day participation in which they can find satisfaction. Public transportation that is limited or unsafe may make group meetings inaccessible to them. The disappearance of certain kinds of hand tools and cooking utensils from the market may make it difficult for them to remain industrious in these domains. A woman laments, "This new apartment came with an electric range and a newfangled microwave oven. I'm too old to learn to cook with such things. So I don't cook at all."

These painful alterations are particularly poignant with respect to the social values discussed earlier, in connection with later-life identity. Many of our elders had looked forward to being respected within their families, for the wisdom and experience accumulated over a lifetime. What some find, instead, is that their personal values concerning daily life differ so much from their children's and grandchildren's that remaining silent is the only way to avoid bitter arguments. Far from being viewed as wise or expert, they feel themselves treated as outmoded and irrelevant. A couple sigh, "Our grandson just got married. They both have fancy taste and fancy plans, and they mean to have it all. When we asked about a baby, he said they won't even think about having a child until they can afford a full-time nanny to raise it. Imagine planning to have children so that you won't have to raise them! Whose children are they anyway? Why have them? We love him so much, and we don't want to hurt him, so we didn't say anything. As long as we keep quiet, he thinks we're sweet and lovable—and rather silly."

In contrast, other people do not experience such differences in values as a challenge to their strong sense of competence. In fact, these differences and the historical and social changes that underlie them seem to serve as a source of wisdom. These fortunate elders are able to call upon a long lifetime of social and political changes to provide empathy and counsel for the younger generations. A woman explains, "I could never give specific advice. They know far more about today's world than I do. But I've been through a lot, and I do know what's right and wrong. I can use my life to help them understand those values, but they have to make their own decisions anyway."

Without exception, the people in our study are able to take pleasure in the accomplishments of their children and grandchildren. In so doing, they seem able to experience a critical measure of vicarious, old-age competence. Several single out for recognition their own attributes and specific areas of expertise, as evidenced in the children. One man proudly says of his son, "He has a drive like mine. He has a lot of push." A couple are proud that all of their children have together taken over the family business and that they are hardworking, efficient, and financially successful. For some people, successes in the next generations reinforce satisfaction in their own achievements. For others, the achievements of children and grandchildren somehow soften disappointment felt at their own failures and inadequacies, both current and past. In particular, those who never completed college invariably take special pride in the degrees earned by children and grandchildren. It seems that they accept some generational responsibility for the sturdy willfulness and steady discipline of the next generations, and that this conspicuous generational success enhances their own sense of lifelong accomplishment and competence.

6. Initiative and Guilt: Purpose

Long after the individual has matured beyond the play age, he or she must continue to temper self-interest and expansiveness with cooperation and concern for others, to exercise disciplined self limitation. These considerations are present in the tension between initiative and guilt in all spheres of life. However, since this tension is ascendant during childhood, when play is a dominant behavioral mode, we regard lifelong expressions of playfulness, throughout the work ethos as well as in recreation and creativity, as particularly relevant to the rebalancing of initiative and guilt. Because this theme is ascendant before socialization subordinates the child's direct sensory perception and expression to cognitive processes that are more linear, we also regard lifelong sensory activity, such as aesthetic appreciation and working with materials, as an important dimension of its reintegration.

The diminution of energy and sensory acuity in old age tempers the elder's participation in the world. Social convention also militates against some overt expression of playfulness. Limited facilities and transportation restrict the kinds of activity that may be readily available. In the face of these age- and society-related obstacles, the individual must rely on a sense of initiative, tempered by a capacity for self-restraint, to renew the strength of purposefulness that was originally developed in childhood. While striving to express initiative through activity, the aged must learn to adapt to new limits on that activity without giving in to incapacitating guilt or overriding inactivation. The elder makes use of current involvement, both to reconcile old-age feelings of initiative and guilt and to integrate a sense of purposefulness that will extend backward and forward, across the whole life cycle.

Virtually all of our informants note that old age brings with it some tendency to let go of the activities and the purposefulness that characterized earlier life. One woman explains, "Of course, you're still interested in everything. But you don't expect yourself to *do* everything, the way you used to. Some things you just have to let go." We have already noted that many people regard these very activities, this very purposefulness, as central to their sense of lifelong identity and industriousness. For them, the later-life struggle to reconcile initiative with guilt and self-limitation is closely linked with efforts to integrate feelings of identity and industriousness that will somehow encompass the entire life cycle. For this reason, this discussion of old-age initiative and guilt will overlap with issues raised in our earlier considerations of identity and identity confusion, and of industry and inferiority.

A wide range of levels of activity reflect our informants' efforts to reconcile activity with inactivation. At one end of the spectrum are those individuals who proudly assert, "You delay aging with activity." These people associate keeping busy with staving off what they view as the physical and emotional ravages of old age. A seventy-nine-year-old woman boasts, "My niece wonders how we have so much energy. How we're always on the go, doing this or that. Well, I say we're just too busy to be sitting around." To this woman, the process of aging seems to connote a stereotyped withdrawal from active involvement with the world at large, in favor of an increasingly reactive preoccupation with personal aches and pains. She views this process as feeding on itself, feeling that if physiological deteriorations are permitted to interfere with activity, they will soon come to dominate life. She explains, "As long as you keep yourself involved in things, you . . . keep your mind occupied so you don't have time to think about yourself or worry about yourself. Once you give in, you're lost." Like many who make a conscious effort to keep busy, this woman equates aging successfully with fighting off, for as long as possible, the inactivation that is currently intolerable but that looms, ultimately, as unavoidable.

The ways in which the elders in our study are able to integrate current enthusiasm and resourcefulness with weary reactiveness must be associated with the ways in which they have reconciled initiative with guilt, since early childhood. Some of those who now make a conscious effort to stay busy describe themselves as having been imaginative and curious as children, as having engaged in assertive, sensory playfulness. From an early age, they were encouraged to play with materials—to draw, to make things, to play music, to garden, to tinker. These people describe having used their senses to explore the world, and they offer still-vivid images of horseback riding on a flourishing family plantation; of smelling the fresh flowers and fruits of a childhood garden; of skating up and down every street of Los Angeles in order to explore the city; of swimming in the sparkling Russian River; of arranging flat stones in a semicircle in a secret clearing in the woods, so the grasses and wildflowers became an audience before whom the subject could recite poems and deliver monologues.

The determinedly active woman noted above has developed a powerful sense of initiative throughout her life cycle. One of her earliest memories is of her grandfather taking a simple piece of paper and, by doing nothing more than folding and cutting, transforming it into a long string of dancing figures. As a child, she delighted in taking simple objects like papers and paintboxes and creating something beautiful, like a picture or a mobile. She recalls a particular incident in which her childhood curiosity about matches led to a small fire on the kitchen's linoleum floor. Notably, she was punished for her dangerously unbridled curiosity in a way that curbed but did not stunt the joy of playful initiative. As an adult, this woman worked for just one employer, shifting jobs as her interest and skill at one task led, inevitably, to something new. She encouraged in her children the same expansive sense of wonder and enthusiasm that she valued in herself. Family activities centered on the out-of-doors, where the children would come to know and understand nature's curious beauties and exhilarating inspirations.

One of this woman's children suffered from a congenital malformation of the heart. Today this malformation is corrected with surgery during infancy. Nearly fifty years ago, however, it was treated by subjecting the patient to an invalid's regime of helplessness and inactivity. Our subject's commitment to the value of energetic exploration, and to the importance of faithful self-reliance, led her to assert herself against conventional medical wisdom, by finding a sympathetic pediatrician and permitting her child to live the "normal" life that she deemed "the only life worth living." She says, "We let her do anything she wanted to do within reason." She recalls that school personnel incessantly sought to arouse her guilt through hysterical phone calls that told her she was going to kill her child. The child's healthy survival reinforced this parent's perpetually renewed sense of purposefulness. As an older woman, she, more than any of our other subjects, conveys a sense of such energetic involvement with diverse aspects of the world that it is difficult to notice the wrinkles in her face or to believe that she is seventy-nine years old. With every gesture, she continues to enact her lifelong philosophy that the world is too full of interesting things to do to waste time "just sitting around."

Near the other end of the spectrum of activity are those elders who seek to dissociate themselves from the idleness they note and criticize in their age-mates—although their own activity levels may be similarly, and unacknowledgedly, low. Apparently unable to come to terms with their own lack of behavioral enterprise, they seek to deny it by voicing no patience for "these people that just sit around. That would be too dull." In particular, our informants disdain the passivity of "senior citizen outings, where they put a bunch of you on a bus and drive you to Tahoe."

Others of our subjects admit that they are getting lazy and

that they let themselves become mesmerized by the television as a way of passing the time. They find themselves withdrawing from longtime club memberships because they no longer feel interested enough to make the effort to attend meetings. The same diminishing interest leads them to lose touch with longtime friends and geographically distant relatives. This tendency leaves some of them feeling uncomfortable and perhaps a little guilty, and they describe it with a note of defensiveness, as does the man who observes, "There is the inclination just to let go . . . to sit here in the evening and watch TV because that is the easiest thing to do. When *you* are over eighty, you'll understand."

Among these individuals are some who describe themselves as having been overly fearful or docile as children. One man recalls, "Curiosity never got me into trouble, because I was always fearful. I always behaved in order to please people." At a time in life when societal institutions rarely demand individual initiative, people like this man may find themselves sinking into guilty passivity. It is not that they choose to remain inactive. Rather, it is that their lifelong sense of initiative has developed in terms of meeting demands that carry the weight of authority. They may have learned to play quietly as children, and even to excel, within a clearly defined set of rules. They may have learned to carry out orders at work, often succeeding creatively within the parameters of a given setting. In the absence of external structures and demands, however, they do not seem to have the capacity to initiate any satisfying activity on their own.

Some of the elders in our study appear to have difficulty coming to terms with the diminished energy of old age. Several describe themselves, today, as far more enterprising and purposeful than their recounted and observable behaviors suggested to the interviewers. One woman calls herself an avid reader, although her home has no books, magazines, or newspapers in evidence and although she cannot remember specific titles or topics of anything she has read recently. Other people speak of themselves as active musicians, photographers, and social entertainers, although they cannot describe a composition they have played or listened to recently, a subject they have photographed, or a guest they have entertained. Perhaps it is a lifelong sense of identity that leads these individuals to continue to think of themselves in terms of activities in which they are no longer able to participate. Perhaps the nature of their integration of initiative and guilt cannot accommodate the changes and limitations that accompany their old age. Unable to acknowledge new limitations, however, they also find themselves unable to develop either new satisfying levels of activity or new internal perceptions of themselves.

Compared with the individuals just discussed, most of the elders in our study are able to integrate more fully their newly depressed levels of enterprise and involvement, and they exemplify a variety of styles of adaptation to what they recognize as the shrinking scope of later life. For example, two women, both in their mid-eighties, report a pronounced absence of the kinds of activity that filled their early retirement days. One says, with matter-of-fact contentment, "We've had most of life's experiences, and we've sort of settled back now to remember and to live out the rest of our life with a great deal of less activity." Admitting a current lack of energy, this woman and her husband become actively involved in recalling and reliving the experiences of a lively past, which came to an end only two or three years ago.

Another reflects a very different kind of adaptation. Speaking slowly, she explains, "I'm old and I won't be here long. I can't do anything any more, but I can give my things to people who will appreciate them." She has given furniture to grandchildren who are setting up their first apartments. She has given favorite paintings and pieces of jewelry to those friends and relatives she associates with each one. Before suffering from a broken arm and arthritis, she had enjoyed painting and making wall hangings from bits of colored glass. Most recently, she contributed all of her materials and the finished work she had lying around to the garage sale a granddaughter was holding to raise money for next year's college expenses. This woman manages to transcend her own current limitations by remaining involved with the people around her through her own belongings. She maintains an active sense of the future, as she gives particular objects away, to individuals who will appreciate them long after she has died.

Most of our informants try to fight the diminished sense of enterprise they anxiously perceive as laziness. In old age, the nature of a satisfying balance between purposeful activity and necessary inactivity may be expected to be different from the equilibrium that was adequate in earlier years. In response to this difference, some of our subjects maintain involvements they value by substituting new variations for specific activities that are now too strenuous. For example, one eighty-year-old has recently found herself unable to continue to serve as a docent at a local art museum. For many years, this woman was a mainstay of the museum's program to introduce fine art to underprivileged elementary school children. She recalls that she used to say that the children kept her young. Now she laughs that they exhausted her into a premature retirement. However, although she no longer has the energy to work with children, she retains her love of art and her interest in the museum with which she has been involved for years. She has translated these ongoing commitments into membership on the research team that gathers background information on the museum's potential acquisitions.

Another woman has long participated in various political activities. She became involved with the League of Women Voters when she and her husband moved into their current house, as new parents. Over the years, she distributed hundreds of thousands of leaflets, door-to-door, and registered hundreds of voters at tables in local shopping centers. However, she eventually became disillusioned with the league's neutrality and redirected her efforts toward partisan politics. Feeling that our times are so precarious that every elected official must count and be held accountable, she actively participated in at least one campaign in each election. In addition, she made a point of supporting all fund-raising activities sponsored by causes she believed in. She baked elaborate cakes for bake sales, brought large casseroles to covered-dish suppers, and quilted bedspreads for raffles. This woman is a victim of rheumatoid arthritis that makes all movement potentially painful. She is still committed to political activism, but she now makes financial, rather than in-kind, contributions to fund-raisers. She acknowledges, "The first time I bought a luncheon ticket instead of bringing one of my special dishes, why, I felt that I was already on the way out. Buying a ticket just wasn't the same as cooking for hours to make a lasagna that would make people drool every time they think of the nuclear freeze. But now I figure that if buying a ticket is the only way I can show support, it's better than sitting home and moping about the good old days."

Several women who once volunteered in such organizations as the Red Cross and the Community Chest now channel their energies into assisting the needy elderly by delivering "meals on wheels," visiting in nursing homes, and knitting for residents of convalescent homes. One woman in her late seventies says, "I am still able to drive, so why shouldn't I deliver these things? You get in contact with people who kind of get you down, but some of them—they just want to talk. They are mostly shut-ins. I feel so sorry for them, and I've always been good at talking to anyone. Society really should involve all these old people in things, though. Get their minds off their worries." One in her nineties says, "I don't want to be home with nothing to do. I may not be able to make my house up nice, and I can't walk anywhere but I forget where I am, but I am still able to knit. I told them I'd use whatever bits of yarn they would give me, and give them back nice warm things for those poor people." For both of these women, this demonstration of old-age initiative is closely tied to the expression of "grand-generativity." They are not simply maintaining lifelong involvements. They are doing so in a fashion that shows sincere and effective concern for others.

The reconciling of later-life initiative with guilt may lead elders, like the woman quoted immediately above, to continue to pursue lifelong avocational involvements in making things. Among such people are those in our study who enjoy gardening and raising exotic ornamental plants; who do woodworking in home workshops; who revamp old cars; who write stories and are assembling autobiographies; who paint and draw; who play musical instruments in small ensembles; and who engage in such fiber crafts as knitting, crocheting, embroidering, beadwork, and decorative sewing. For all of these individuals, the maintaining of longtime avocations is often a struggle. Their participation is often more erratic and occasionally more indirect than they would like. However, they concur that they derive real satisfaction from continuing to "make something special and beautiful like a sweater out of something ordinary like wool."

Other people are able to find in old age an opportunity to develop new kinds of involvement with the world of doing and making. As was discussed earlier, one woman is in the process of remodeling and redecorating her home. Although she does not physically do the painting or carpentry, she plans and directs every move the workmen make. Demonstrating considerable executive and evaluative capacity, she gives the impression of relishing the inevitable fretting in which this infinite series of small projects constantly involves her. This woman has never worked with wood or paint, and she has not begun to do so now. However, in deciding to undertake this remodeling, she has begun to be successfully involved, albeit indirectly, with a kind of project she has long admired and of which she has long been afraid.

For some of the elders in our study, working with their hands was a primary vocation. These individuals are among the few who have been able to remain purposefully involved in the area of primary vocational commitment, even after retirement and into old age. They may experience a close connection between the lifelong strength of purpose that is related to recreation, and the sense of competence that is an integral part of work. One such person is the Sierra foothills rancher, discussed in earlier sections, who has now turned the ranch over to his children. Although he has relinquished official responsibility, he still lives on the land and works in the fields and the orchards because he loves to do so—as he always has. He laughingly observes that he now has trouble differentiating work from play. Purposeful, work-related activities have for him remained a source of pleasure well into later life.

Among our informants are ones who have always used their senses in active aesthetic appreciation. They have eagerly attended the theater and the opera; they have visited and volunteered in museums. They have encouraged their friends who paint and have enthusiastically admired their work. However, in old age they experience constraints on the kinds of aesthetic activities they can engage in. One of these people can no longer drive to the opera. Another's wife can no longer sit still through a full-length theater production. A third cannot walk through more than one room of a museum without stopping for a long rest. On the basis of initiative and purposefulness that have developed since childhood, many of these people resourcefully take advantage of home-based facsimiles of the outside activities they now find inaccessible. They use television as a source of opera and theater; they appreciate works of art in library books. Some even respond to limitations with ingenuity that overcomes inaccessibility itself. For example, the woman who tires after being on her feet for a short period has begun to arrange for wheelchairs, rather than relinquish the pleasure of going to museums.

Demonstrating enterprise and taking advantage of opportunity, several elders seem to come into their own in old age, in ways that have hitherto eluded them. A woman who has long viewed herself as a failed artist has recently begun to do cartooning. This woman has always highly prized artistic talent and success. Her early work did not meet with instant acclaim, and she did not push her talent to its limits. Instead of pursuing a graduate degree in fine arts or a career as a painter, she succumbed to her parents' edict that painting was not nearly as valuable as marrying. She married and devoted her middle-adult life to raising five children, managing a financially strained household, and providing emotional support for her husband. She expressed her artistic inclinations in the ways she arranged the family's succession of homes, the pillows and tapestries she made, the ways she painted the children's rooms, and the kinds of clothes she made for other family members. Now, living in an age-restricted setting, she has begun to draw cartoons of old people living in retirement communities. For her, cartooning seems to be a lively, imaginative transformation of experience. It is an ingenious way to turn encroaching helplessness and debilitation into something creative and enjoyable, as well as a potential source of acclamation from her peers.

In our discussion of retirement, we noted that separation from the work setting often removes the individual from those circumstances in which he or she learned to demonstrate competence and initiative. Thus, retirement may leave the elder without the structure that has come to be essential, or at least customary, in behaving with skillfulness and creativity. The life of the following informant, however, suggests that this dynamic does not hold true for individuals who have retired from jobs they regarded as boring and stifling. This widowed man lives alone in a cabin in a sparsely populated, rural area. Throughout his working career, he held a variety of low-paying jobs that, in retrospect, neither required nor permitted real discipline or enterprise. He did not particularly like his jobs, and he was never viewed as performing them with particular success. For this man, retirement seems to signify not the loss of valuable structure, but his release from a series of rigid, repetitive demands that in and of themselves precluded inventiveness and enthusiasm. Retirement presents him with a new opportunity to reexperience the initiative that he now recalls as having characterized him until his midteens.

This man has always enjoyed music. He has always loved listening to the radio and playing records. As an adolescent, he tinkered with radio equipment until the advent of transistors and integrated circuits. Over the years he has accumulated a collection of some two to three thousand 78 rpm records. Recognizing that plastic record disks are likely to warp or break, he has recently begun to copy them onto cassettes. He has removed his tape deck and large loudspeakers from their cabinet and strapped them to a mover's dolly, onto which he has built appropriate shelves. Each day, when he goes to the senior center for lunch, he wheels his movable entertainment center out to his pickup truck and brings his friends their favorite songs. This man has also begun to make his own TV dinners, using the partitioned trays on which his "meals on wheels" are delivered. He cooks large quantities of meat and vegetables and freezes them in these single-meal trays for easy access. The quality of this man's products is far from professional. In fact, his entertainment center looks rather slapdash, and the contents of his frozen meals do not always retain flavor or texture when reheated. What is striking, instead, is the enthusiasm, the delight, and the pride with which he has devised his various projects. In each case he perceived a problem, combined his own ingenuity with the resources at hand to devise a solution that is satisfactory for his own needs, and created something that is usable, gives him pleasure, and remains a real source of personal pride.

Other subjects do not seem to be able to sustain a sense of purpose in the face of the guilt and anxiety elicited by the internal or external limitations of old age. Although they may say they have enjoyed art and music throughout adulthood, in the weariness of old age they find themselves unable to seize the aesthetic opportunities that do exist. For example, one woman complains bitterly of missing the symphony. She lives alone and cannot drive at night. In addition, back problems make it difficult for her to stay seated for more than twenty or thirty minutes. Her son has begun to give her records of the compositions performed at the symphony series she used to attend. But although she is touched by his concern, she somehow has not managed to play even one of these records. Perhaps this woman's enjoyment of the symphony was so closely tied to the excitement of spending an evening among the other music lovers at symphony hall that the music, alone, promises to be lifeless. For her, playing a record at home may vividly symbolize her age-related limitations; by not playing the records she may be seeking to avoid confronting these limitations.

Some informants express profound regret at having relinquished such activities as painting, singing, playing music, and photography. In a way that we find puzzling, these individuals do not seem to be able to explain why they abandoned meaningful involvements in the first place, or why they have failed to find new, more satisfying ones in their stead. They seem to want to believe that they gave up long-cherished activities because circumstances forced them to do so and that these same circumstantial constraints have prevented them from adopting substitutes. But the circumstances they mention do not appear to be convincingly constraining. A woman whose life is relatively free of daily commitments laments that she has stopped playing the piano because she simply cannot find the time. A photographer explains that he no longer takes pictures, because he cannot muster the energy to invite friends to view his slides. Experiencing difficulty in balancing accustomed enthusiasm with increasing ennui, these people seem to be enacting a conflict between a tendency to decrease their level of creative activity and an unsettling sense of guilt at doing so without justifiable, external reasons. Unable to understand or accept their current behavior, they are struggling to ascribe it to external causes.

Several of the elders in our study devote considerable time

and energy to corresponding with long-distance friends and relatives they have known, in some cases, for more than sixty years. Many count this mode of visiting with the people they love among their most enjoyable ways of spending time. These people were not always letter writers. They did not predict that they would enjoy this activity in old age. But they currently find themselves unable to sustain any other form of meaningful contact. They cannot drive long distances. They have neither the physical nor the financial stamina for long trips by air. So they have learned to communicate through the mails. They may exchange photographs, newspaper clippings, and poems. They may write short notes or long, thoughtful, wandering letters. All of these styles of correspondence represent ways these individuals have adapted to the shrinking horizons of old age without relinquishing the most important of life's activities.

For some of the elders with whom we spoke, it seems that grandparenthood makes possible the expression of a kind of initiative that might otherwise not have overcome existing apathy or hesitancy. The faces of these people light up as they describe visits and outings with grandchildren. One man eagerly notes, "Rather than buy things for myself, or go to the movies or suchlike, I spend my money to bring the grandchildren down to visit." This kind of enthusiasm is particularly striking in those individuals who seem to display little real interest in other aspects of current life.

A wrinkled, white-haired woman smiles and says, "I do things with the grandchildren that I'd never do without them. Just silly little things that make you feel so good!" This woman acknowledges an occasional temptation to stay up until all hours, giggling with a friend, or to walk in the rain for the sheer pleasure of being outside and being wet. But according to social convention, old people who engage in

such activity may be questioned about the age appropriateness of their behavior. And she, like many of our subjects,
is quite mindful of social judgment. "I don't really care what
they think," she says. "But I'm not so quick as I once was
to thumb my nose at them. When you get to be my age, you
don't want to offend someone you may need to rely on."
Concern for social propriety is a necessary part of the equilibrium, established in earliest childhood, between an expansive
sense of playfulness and initiative and a limiting sense of
guilt. This concern continues to play a role in the integration
of initiative and guilt, throughout the life cycle, perhaps
wielding its greatest influence in those periods during which
the individual holds least social power and can muster least
personal confidence. Old age is, arguably, one such period.
Anticipatory guilt over potential misconduct leads a number
of our subjects to curb a certain amount of their playfulness
and curiosity. Sharing such behaviors with grandchildren,
however, is regarded as another, far more acceptable matter.
Thus, it is with grandchildren that many elders most freely
and enthusiastically express the spontaneity that is deemed
inappropriate in so many of the other settings and with so
many of the other people who are part of an old person's
daily life.

Our informants express curiosity about and involvement
with the world at large in a number of different ways. Some
say they watch television to keep abreast of things going on
in the world. Many subscribe to newspapers and magazines
in order to remain informed about current events. Others
read in a more disciplined fashion, choosing topics of interest
and actively seeking books on those topics. One woman has
become quite knowledgeable about world religions and their
cultural origins. Another has learned a good deal about early
American textiles and silver. One retired chemical engineer

meets with a group from the university department of chemistry to discuss the kinds of theoretical and research ideas that the more applied orientation of his career did not offer him the time to pursue.

For many elders, travel seems to be a vehicle for giving free play to curiosity and the urge to explore, for testing personal limits in unfamiliar settings. Several of our subjects have used retirement as an opportunity to begin to see places they had hitherto only dreamed about. Some have made worldwide trips. Others have made frequent shorter trips by car. In all of these cases, the traveling experience seems to have been permeated with the spirit of adventure that is inherent in initiative throughout the life cycle. Among our informants, those who still travel, who look forward to going to visit distant relatives or to taking trips for pleasure, seem, as a whole, to express far more of a sense of involvement in day-to-day possibilities than do those who relegate their traveling to the past.

A number of our informants find themselves struggling to adjust to a new partner or a new home. Such adjustment may activate feelings of inventiveness and of weariness as well. In so doing, it is a catalyst for their reexperiencing; that is, it provides an arena for an essential reassessment that might otherwise be deferred. In new relationships, with or without legal confirmation, elders find themselves assuming new partnership responsibilities and developing new daily routines, new ways of living, new activities, and new opportunities—all of which require exploration and creative accommodation if satisfactory adaptation is to be made. As in earlier-life relationships, elders find themselves testing the strength of their own purposefulness, in comparison with the limits and wishes of their partners. One remarried woman struggling with new frustration says, "In my first marriage

I did everything at home. He had none of those responsibilities at all, and I don't know if he could have made a bed or
washed a meal's worth of dishes if his life depended on it. I
don't want to do that again, and I was determined that this
marriage would be different. My new husband lived alone
after his first wife died, so I know he knows how to do things
at home. But I guess he assumes that the household is the
wife's responsibility. Sometimes I am determined not to give
in. Other times I just don't have the energy to disagree."

Similar kinds of exploration and imagination are required
of those who move to new homes in old age. These people
struggle as they enact accustomed territoriality and lifelong
routine, on the one hand, and reluctant weariness to set up
all over again, on the other. This struggle takes place in a new
physical context, which carries its own conventions and im-
poses its own limits.

As the elders in our study look back on a lifetime of
gratifying activity and self-limiting inactivity, a number of
them ruminate about initiative missed or failed, and they
dwell excessively on feelings of guilt over specific instances
of initiative *not* taken. One man failed to act at the critical
moment of choice concerning his marriage, and he is plagued
by seventy-year-old images of a train from which he did not
have the courage to disembark. Another never pursued a
career in writing, although in his own eyes and those of his
family, his literary talent had distinguished him early and
although he had been planning to become a writer for as long
as he could remember. In old age, neither of these men can
see beyond perceived critical failures and passivity to appreciate the purposefulness they have also demonstrated. As if
to compensate for unseized opportunity, one daydreams
about "gambling and hitting the jackpot right and left." Both
find themselves spending many of their waking hours ac-

tively regretting their missed initiative and disdaining the bored listlessness they see in their peers—and try not to see in themselves. The ways these individuals are guiltily tied to the past make it difficult for them to demonstrate in the present the initiative that is essential for a satisfying lifelong sense of purpose.

In no stage of life are people able to undo action taken or not taken in the past. What they may reasonably expect, however, is to acknowledge past experiences of initiative and guilt and to participate in purposeful involvements, in the present, that facilitate the integrating of these lifelong tendencies, while the opportunity remains to do so. One woman explains, "I don't dwell on the things I did wrong. There were plenty. I lived my life as best I could, and I still do, and that's all I can do at this point."

7. AUTONOMY AND SHAME/DOUBT: WILL

The tension between autonomy and shame/doubt involves very early issues of control over one's own body, one's own behavior, and, in a larger sense, one's own life. Once, as a toddler, the individual has established basic control over sphincter and skeletal muscles, he or she spends a lifetime struggling to balance the exercise of will with discriminating self-restraint—to be independent and true to oneself, and simultaneously to be concerned with safety and convention. As the body changes and develops throughout the life cycle, capacities for autonomous behavior also develop and change, expanding and contracting with the overall waxing and waning of physical prowess. Along with actual behavioral capacities, individual feelings of self-determination and of helplessness remain connected with the body, and they resurface

throughout life—at times, for example, of bodily damage
from illness or injury, of the bodily changes of puberty, and
of the deteriorations of old age.

With the failing physical capacities associated even with
the healthiest aging, the limits of personal autonomy undergo an inevitable constriction. The elder has known the
fullest extent of physical self-reliance as well as adulthood's
greatest measure of willful mastery over other aspects of life.
In old age, he or she confronts limitations that are both
internal and external in origin, related to actual physical
capacity, and also to societal stereotype and expectation. In
the face of new limitations, the elder must struggle to maintain the willfulness and the independence that remain possible. This struggle, like those surrounding the other themes
discussed thus far, comprises the observable realm of behavior and the related, more private realm of feelings. The people in our study strive to maintain behavioral adequacy,
despite increasing physical disability. They endeavor to remain independent, despite increasing needs for various kinds
of assistance. In an effort to balance stubborness with compliance, they seek to make some kind of personal peace with
societal expectations of the aged, without surrendering the
sense of self-determination that is essential to the sense of
autonomy throughout the life cycle.

Almost all of our informants suffer from one or another
of a vast array of old-age-related physiological and psycho
logical disorders, which, like those in the aged population as
a whole, range from a simple diminution of earlier capacities
to conditions that seriously impair day-to-day functioning.
Regardless of the *degree* of functional impact, each disorder
has a qualitative functional impact that influences the individual's equilibration of the opposing tendencies toward autonomy and toward shame or doubt. Even those people who

describe themselves as being in excellent health and in no way physically limited nonetheless observe that they tire more easily than in earlier life and that they simply do not have the energy to do all of the things they used to do. Most of them mention impaired vision or hearing, often corrected with eyeglasses and hearing aids. These simple impairments necessitate an ongoing dependence on corrective procedures and devices.

The woman who needs a nap after two hours of driving around town can no longer decide, spontaneously, to drop in on a friend for lunch after completing a morning's errands. If she schedules her time carefully, and if traffic obliges, she may be able to run errands and enjoy a social lunch on the same morning. But she must plan in advance, and even then her plans may not work out. While this diminished capacity and others like it do not necessarily detract from behavioral adequacy, they complicate the comings and goings of old age, and they necessitate change in the individual's middle-adulthood sense of near-absolute, willful control over the activities of daily life.

Many of our informants have difficulty in moving, as a result of arthritis, acute illness, or incomplete recuperation from bruises, broken bones, or surgery; two are confined to wheelchairs. Several mention such chronic ailments as heart disease, high blood pressure, and undiagnosed coughing— often accompanied by a history of heavy smoking—although few of these are either life-threatening or wholly disabling. A few elders note digestive disorders like ulcers and fistulas, uncontrollable gagging, and difficulties in swallowing. Several either describe or display some degree of cognitive difficulty, ranging from annoying memory losses to pervasive thought disorders. While these multifarious impairments can limit activity, the degree to which they do so is influenced by the individual's lifelong experience of self-determination. Several rather severely disabled persons acknowledge the realistic limitations imposed by their disabilities, while engaging in the activities that are still possible and developing appropriate, new, self-directed involvements. These individuals do not permit physiological deterioration to restrict the scope of their lives any more than is absolutely necessary. Relying on a sense of willfulness developed throughout the life cycle, they renew a robust sense of willfulness in old age.

The following two women in their late eighties exemplify assertive accommodation to disability, based on a lifelong, vigorous sense of autonomy. The first, suffering from painful arthritis and from chemically and surgically treated ulcerations throughout her digestive tract, moved from her rural home a year after her husband's death, because by herself she could no longer maintain their two-acre fruit-and-vegetable garden. Although accepting this restriction, she took an apartment in an intergenerational complex in a small urban area. Setting up her new home involved making friends with her new neighbors, putting in a patio garden, and scouting out the local commercial areas so that she could combine necessary shopping with the walking she was determined to do each day. This woman has never enjoyed housekeeping, and she admits, "If I were in better condition, I might keep my house cleaner, but probably not." For those physical activities in which she cannot (and will not) engage, she has substituted increased reading about historical cultures and world religions, writing short stories and vignettes, which she submits for journal publication, and working on an autobiography for her grandchildren. Physiological disabilities have resulted in major changes in this woman's day-to-day activities. But she continues to assert her independence, choosing from among the possible activities those that are personally meaningful.

The second woman to be considered here suffers from many seriously disabling conditions. An inveterate smoker and a diabetic, she has had one leg amputated and is confined to a wheelchair. She has a chronic heart condition and kidney and bladder trouble. Bad circulation indicates that she may soon lose her second leg to surgery. Not too long ago, she underwent major surgeries on her gall bladder, rectum, reproductive system, and varicose veins. In addition, she is legally blind and her hearing is deteriorating.

This woman lives with the family of her youngest daughter —the youngest of six children and four stepchildren. She readily acknowledges that she cannot live on her own, that she cannot reliably perform the many householding tasks that have been associated with her identity throughout adulthood, and that she cannot wholly care for herself or meet her own needs within her daughter's family. She sorely misses her once-enjoyed activities, particularly reading and cooking. She does not like her unavoidable dependence on her daughter, son-in-law, and grandchildren. Such realistic behavioral helplessness is more than likely to induce feelings of shameful inadequacy. However, this woman continues to demonstrate autonomy, in the ways she participates both in social interaction and in solitary, self-directed activities. For example, although she is legally blind and might be expected to be largely reactive in conversation, she takes advantage of the visual cues she is able to perceive, and she engages her companions as fully as possible. Smilingly aware of the flattery involved, she explained to the interviewer, "I can't see myself in the mirror to tell if my lipstick is on straight. I can't tell what color your eyes are, but I can see what shape you are and how you move. I can tell that your hair is long and pulled back, and I can certainly tell that you are young and pretty. So that tells me how to talk to you."

Unable to rely on her eyes, this inveterate reader now makes liberal use of talking books. She is never far from her tape recorder, and she sometimes enjoys "dirty books—books that would have shocked [her] generation." Although she is unable to be responsible for housecleaning tasks or meal preparation, she does not hesitate to act on impulse in these areas. "If I want to bake a cake during the day, I just do it," she says. "I get tired, reaching up to the counter from my wheelchair, but I can do it if I take my time and put my mind to it." To counteract the feelings of loneliness and isolation that often result from wheelchair confinement accompanied by serious sensory impairment, this woman carries a portable radio with her at all times. "I even take my radio to bed with me," she notes. "They give all the news, and I try to keep knowing about the world. I try to get as much out of life as I can."

Both of the women just discussed have adjusted to realistic limitations, while continuing to exercise those forms of self-reliance that remain possible. Although they both hint at being somewhat ashamed of their increasing dependence, they have been able to rely on strong, lifelong willfulness in their old-age efforts tenaciously to preserve an essential sense of their own autonomy. Both are actively struggling to limit the extent to which impairment results in "disability," an inability to perform activity normally, or in "handicap," an inability to fulfill role functions.* For both of these women, the dynamic, resilient balance between a sense of autonomy

---

*S. J. Brody, "Is Rehabilitation a Legitimate Intervention for the Elderly? Goals and Expectations," in C. M. Gaitz, G. Niederehe, and N. L. Wilson, eds., *Aging 2000: Our Health Care Destiny,* vol. 2, *Psychosocial and Policy Issues* (New York: Springer Verlag, 1985), 237–47.

and feelings of shame and doubt has kept the impairment from leading to the disability and the handicap that are often associated with old age. They demonstrate that although impairment and a certain degree of disability may be inevitable in old age, handicap and its deleterious effects on psychosocial well-being need not necessarily follow.

In striking contrast, other elders in our study seem to succumb to feelings of uncertainty, concerning both their capacities and their impression on others. Their more fragile or brittle lifelong will to assert themselves now appears to be broken in response to physiological limitations. They allow impairments and disabilities to impose on activity and independence generalized constrictions that do not seem to be necessitated by physiological conditions, in and of themselves.

One woman in her early nineties, afflicted with pervasive arthritis, admits that although she is able to walk, she is so afraid of falling that she moves as little as possible. She explains, "I'm not so much afraid of getting hurt. But what would it look like—a grown woman falling all over herself like a two-year-old?" For this woman, social appropriateness has always been an important component of the way autonomy comes into scale with shame and doubt. Ever conscious of her image as a proper, well-raised woman, she has always chosen activities in order to enhance that image. She was a stalwart member of the Eastern Star and the community garden club, participating with special pride in the evening receptions and afternoon teas, for which she could wear the long gowns and flowing dresses in which she had always felt most feminine. She dressed her young daughters in ruffles and frills, and she is proud of how beautifully they now dress their own children. Her arthritis makes it impossible for her to move gracefully or with confidence. Although she might still attend the functions she has always enjoyed, she does not feel she could do so with the elegance she views as necessary to her image. Even faltering in the privacy of her own home is a potential source of embarrassment. She determines her behavior not in order to maximize functional participation but in order to minimize the embarrassment that represents such a threat to her sense of autonomy.

Among our informants, it does not seem to be the particular physical capacity or incapacitation itself that most strongly affects the old-age integration of feelings of autonomy with those of shame and doubt. Rather, it is the *meaning* of an experienced disability—and such meaning varies widely from person to person. The ability or inability to continue to drive, directly associated with visual and reflex impairment, is a good example. For some individuals, "it was the hardest thing in the world to give up the freedom of driving." These people clung to that freedom as long as they possibly could, and they seem to regard its forced relinquishment as a shameful personal loss. For others, failing vision and slowed reflexes, even within acceptable legal limits, had transformed driving into a frightening activity or an experience of embarrassing incompetence. When one such man gave his car to his daughter, the act of giving represented a behavior, unlike driving, in which he could still engage with autonomous pleasure and pride. His sense of later-life independence is enhanced by his having removed himself from the dangerous, humiliating experience of driving badly, in a fashion that also showed generative concern for his daughter. This enhancement brings into scale his more painful feelings of embarrassment and helplessness.

For those elders who choose to forgo driving by giving the car to a younger relative, the bequest often carries with it the expectation that necessary transportation will be provided for them, that their mobility will no longer depend on their own, increasingly inconsistent capacities. For these people, mobility reliably provided by others seems to represent greater autonomy than the unreliable mobility they are able to provide for themselves. These individuals have been able to acknowledge realistic doubt about their driving abilities and to continue to express autonomy in making gifts and in accepting assistance that increases the radius in which they can participate in self-chosen activities. They have come to experience autonomy in new ways and, in so doing, to accept with dignity certain kinds of assistance that would earlier have signified intolerable helplessness.

It is not only the personal meaning of any given ability or disability that influences an elder's readjusted sense of independence and self-respect. Society also attaches to such abilities meanings that profoundly affect feelings of personal assertiveness, self-reliance, and embarrassment. To continue with the example of driving a car, in contemporary American life this activity represents both a realistic source of convenient, efficient transportation and an expression of individual independence. As one of our cultural rites of passage into adulthood, driving also seems to signify a clear membership in adult society. In many states, numerous financial and professional transactions require a valid driver's license as a form of personal identification. For all such transactions, the mere lack of a driver's license may well handicap an old person's performance of such adulthood privileges as paying for purchases by check, cashing a check, or maintaining financial credit. In such terms, an age-related inability to continue to drive necessitates the relinquishing not only of convenience and self-directed mobility but also of some measure of commercial independence and of social adulthood. That is, the voluntary, realistic relinquishing of one form of autonomy seems to be tied to the involuntary, unnecessary relinquishing of other forms as well.

The expression and experience of willfulness are related not just to the elder's attitudes toward specific abilities but also to feelings about overall physical health. Many of our informants describe themselves—some proudly, some more matter-of-factly—as being strong and healthy for their age. That these descriptions are based on psychological as well as physiological reality is suggested by the wheelchair-bound woman discussed above, who is included among these self-identified, "healthier than average" individuals. She explains, "I'm very healthy; my leg is very sick."

To many of these people, a sense of autonomous well-being seems to be so closely tied to a diagnosis of better-than-average health that they provide such diagnoses themselves, in the presence or absence of professional corroboration. Some simply do not mention current medical disorders unless explicitly asked—even when such disorders are chronic and may require repeated hospitalization. Instead, they speak of the importance of being independent and describe their current lives in terms of the self-reliance and functional independence they are able to maintain. For example, in our first interview one woman avowed her determination, "come hell or high water," to remain in the community in which she manages quite well on her own: "I know the shops and the streets and the neighbors. And I know my way around this little apartment. I keep myself fed, clothed, and happy—and that's pretty good for an old gal like me. Of course, I've always been able to count on being strong and healthy." Only in the second interview, scheduled with some difficulty after the informant had failed to answer several phone calls and a letter from the interviewer, did this woman mention the condition for which she had been hospitalized during the entire period between our two interviews. This was the third surgery she had recently undergone for what she describes as near-chronic intestinal bleeding.

Some of our subjects actively deny pervasive disabilities, as if the asserting of heroic willfulness could make generalized self-reliance a reality. In so doing, they cut themselves off from potentially valuable medical or therapeutic assistance. One woman, in her middle eighties and nearly crippled with arthritis throughout her body, is a good example. Long characterized by determination, she now insists that she will not use a wheelchair but, instead, will go anywhere she wants to go on her own steam, walking with a cane. However, because she cannot walk assisted only by a cane, she rarely moves beyond her bed, bathroom, and breakfast bar. She seems to regard her realistic inability to walk as an intolerable humiliation, and she will not acknowledge it. Unable to accept the wheelchair, which she apparently considers a *symbol* of helplessness, she seems, instead, to have succumbed to real helplessness. This woman readily acknowledges her impaired condition; it is the resulting disability that she denies. And the denial of disability, while it shows bravado, seems to have resulted in unnecessary handicap.

In reviewing physical health across the entire life cycle, a number of the people in our study deny the existence of longitudinally documented, chronic pathologies from earlier life. The self-image of lifelong robust health seems to be so indispensable to these individuals' sense of autonomy in old age that they do not admit their past illnesses. For example, one man describes a variety of current orthopedic disorders, exacerbated by an almost fatal virus he contracted two years ago in the rural Far East. This man, now in his mid-eighties, emphasizes his efforts to overcome his ailments and not to let them interfere with his activity: "I have always been healthy, and I am not used to restriction. I have always been a very active person in my work, in sports, and in all forms of recreation with the family. Until this business with my joints, that is." He speaks wistfully of missing the bicycling, skating, skiing, and driving that his hips and ankles will no longer permit. It is striking that he consistently fails to acknowledge the serious hypotension and accompanying cardiac arrhythmia, which, according to historical data, forced him to discontinue many of these activities as long as four or five decades ago. Like those people mentioned earlier whose current sense of autonomy requires that they see themselves as extraordinarily healthy, this man provides the retroactive diagnosis of good physical health that his current psychological well-being seems to demand.

Not all of our informants deny either specific disabilities or the expectable deterioration of old age. Most wistfully acknowledge, "Old people miss having strength. You want to do, and know you need help." What varies is the level to which they are able to personalize this acknowledgment— that is, the extent to which they can integrate feelings of shame and resignation with the autonomous stance that is socially and personally more acceptable. Some speak of the humiliation of friends and spouses who find themselves failing. Some frankly discuss these matters using the all-inclusive *we*. A few even manage to speak directly of themselves. However personal or impersonal the pronouns, most of the people in our study express understandable regret at lost capacities and new weaknesses. Some express anger: "You watch yourself gradually deteriorate, and it makes you mad. Old age is cruel." Nearly all articulate the wish to die before becoming "a real basket case."

Thus far we have indicated that our subjects demonstrate

widely varying levels of integration of realistic physiological deterioration. In contrast, they openly express an almost unanimous fear of mental deterioration. A coronary patient says, "I'm lucky to have my brains." A Meals on Wheels volunteer observes, "I forget things, and that does scare me." Many voice a terror of losing their mind, speaking so quickly as to suggest superstitious avoidance of the very words. Most assert, "I don't want to linger. No rest home. No convalescent home. I don't want to go on living one minute after I'm mentally incapable." To all of these people, apparently, physiological disability can be compensated for or denied in the service of willful autonomy. But a disabled mind can neither deny nor compensate. In its most profound sense, then, mental disability seems to loom as a shameful helplessness that will permit no vestiges of autonomy, in the realm either of behavior or of internal feelings.

Although many of the elders in our study note the importance of having good health in old age, relatively few speak in a way that indicates active, conscious responsibility for maintaining optimal physical well-being through exercise and diet. Among these exceptions is one hardworking couple who extol the health-related values of physical labor. Though formally retired, these people still rise early and, following their own advice, continue to work hard in their lifelong business, maintaining their own stamina and speaking with a combination of concern and disapproval of their peers who sit around, waiting to be cared for. A few individuals rather halfheartedly mention doing some form of regular exercise, such as walking, golfing, or going through an exercise routine.

One woman describes being scrupulously careful about her diet, in order to remain healthy enough to do the folk dancing to which she is passionately devoted. To her way of

thinking, self-discipline in her cooking enables her to preserve the good health that is essential if she is to continue to
dance. That is, one form of self-directed behavior permits
this woman to maintain the involvement that she regards as
absolutely essential to her overall independent survival. Enthusiastically, she explains, "You can conquer it [old age's
debilitation] if you really want to." In fact, the physical
activity she strives to maintain itself makes a contribution to
the health that is integral to her sense of autonomy.

Living independently seems to be a very important symbol
of autonomy for our informants, and most of them are living
under circumstances they perceive as independent. Even
though the maintaining of longtime dwellings and routines
has become impossible for many, these people seem to experience freedom and self-reliance in sharing a home with a
socially acceptable, more independent "roommate," or in
living alone with outside assistance—in protected retirement
communities or in partial-care facilities that comprise individual residential units. The capacities to behave with self-
reliance and to experience a sense of autonomy are often
closely tied not only to living independently but also to living
in familiar surroundings and carrying out well-established
routines. In such a supportive environment, elders can feel
confident in facing encroaching inadequacies and doubts
with whatever autonomy is still realistic. Without these familiar supports, inadequacies, limitations, and humiliations
can seem potentially overwhelming.

However, for some of the people in our study, maintaining
such self-determination often conflicts with securing the assistance they and their families recognize as increasingly
necessary. In particular, elders' longtime residences are often
quite a distance from the relatives our informants depend on
for assistance. For example, upon returning home from a

relatively brief hospitalization, a woman who has always been proud of her strong-willed independence found herself deliberating, "I know it would be so much more convenient for them [in the next generation] if I lived nearer, but I'm just not ready to move. I don't want to be a burden out here, and I guess sometimes I am. I just like my independence." To paraphrase her rumination and those of many others, "The life I know how to live is *here*. If I leave, I'll *really* be helpless."

In an earlier section, we discussed the ways in which the intergenerational exchange of advice and assistance seems to express a dimension of our informants' old-age reintegration of the tension between generative caring and stagnant self-centeredness. Various aspects of this exchange are also related to the struggle to balance independence and self-reliance with dependence and shame. A corollary of the often-quoted assertion "No man is an island" is the observation that we all need various forms of advice and assistance, as each of us makes his or her own way through life. In old age, as distinct from earlier life, our informants find themselves requiring assistance with a plethora of tasks they had hitherto performed without a second thought. One man in his seventies can no longer plow his own vegetable fields or chop all of his own wood for the winter. Unless he receives assistance, he can neither plant the large garden that regularly supplies him and his neighbors with fresh produce nor keep his wood stove burning throughout the winter. One woman in her nineties cannot reach up high, and she has had to ask for help reorganizing her kitchen in order to store necessary dishes and pots within reach. Both of these people have been able to view necessary assistance as supplementary to their own efforts. For them, the balancing of realistic helplessness and embarrassment with longstanding willfulness and assertiveness has involved coming to regard assistance as facilitating overall autonomy rather than as threatening or substituting for personal independence. To the man, growing his own vegetables and living in his own cabin are important expressions of autonomy. To the woman, continuing to cook for herself in her own apartment represents independence. Both of them are able to accept assistance as a necessary component of their maintaining this autonomy and independence.

By comparison, other elders demonstrate a more rigidly defined sense of self-reliance, according to which requiring assistance of any kind represents a shameful failure of autonomy. The accomplishment of specific, unassisted activities has become an end in itself, rather than serving as a means toward a goal. For example, a woman in her eighties was temporarily confined to a wheelchair with a broken knee. Her home has a lovely sunken entryway, which features four flower-lined steps descending from the street to the front door and another two steps descending from the level of the front hall and bedrooms, into the living room. She and her husband needed the efforts of two strong men to lift the wheelchair, every time she wanted to go outside or into the living room. Looking back on the way they handled that circumstance, she says, "We have always prided ourselves on our independence. It felt so awful to have to send for help every time I left the house and came back that I just didn't leave at all, except to go to the doctor. Nothing we would do outside was important enough to make it worth feeling so helpless. A club meeting or a movie or a dinner with friends —or even playing the piano in the living room. Not worth feeling helpless for. So I pretty much stayed in the bedroom and watched TV. But I did it on my own."

Some of our informants are members of communities in

which individuals help one another both on a personal level and in an organized, communitywide fashion. For example, in one rural area the man who was driving all of his friends to the senior center and to the nearest desirable stores found that his truck had become too small for all of his prospective passengers. That group of elders organized to buy and maintain their own van; those who still drive take turns at the wheel.

Some of our subjects hire people to perform such services as gardening, housecleaning, and housekeeping, as well as personal care, both for themselves and for disabled family members. For those who can afford it, the hiring of assistance —independently employing a worker—seems to represent a self-directed way of securing necessary services without surrendering autonomy. In contrast, the relying on assistance from relatives can represent embarrassingly dependent helplessness. One woman explains, "I'll never lose my independence. No matter what I might not be able to do for myself, I will never have to rely on the goodwill of anybody, because I can always pay for whatever I might ever need."

Some of our informants provide assistance to other people as an important component of self-direction and independence, a valuable counterweight to acknowledged elements of dependence. As we discussed in an earlier chapter, this process is often a component of generative care as well. Several elders are either now engaged in caring for a seriously disabled spouse or sibling or have been so in the past. One extremely self-reliant woman in her midseventies notes that two of her siblings have recently moved nearby so that she can keep an eye on them. Although she is somewhat critical of their need for her, her ability to be helpful to them certainly confirms her lifelong sense of herself as reliable, energetic, and independent.

For most of the people in our study, a request for help seems to show an uncomfortable deficiency, whereas the offer and provision of assistance indicate a comparative adequacy. However, even this feeling of adequacy is not reassuring in all circumstances. Think back to the man discussed earlier, with respect to old-age intimacy and isolation, who cares at home for his almost wholly incapacitated wife. While his own relative strength and physical integrity reinforce some aspects of his sense of personal autonomy, the extent to which he remains tied to a frightened invalid seriously constrains the freedom that constitutes another aspect of independence in later life. In addition, this man knows that he cannot depend on his lifelong partner as he experiences and mourns his own deterioration. His ability to keep his wife out of an institution today does not provide the reassurance that he so desperately wants, that in his own very old age someone will do the same for him.

Many of our informants depend on the goodwill of their children to give necessary assistance. In general, they derive a sense of autonomy from knowing that their children will keep them independent of more bureaucratic, institutionalized services. Even those who pay for some kinds of household assistance are pleased to rely on their children for interim housing and storage, for moral support, and for advice. This intergenerational dependence often seems to strengthen a sense of the generational cycle. It also seems to create in our subjects a feeling of security that serves as a critical foundation for overall autonomy. This dynamic is reminiscent of the process through which a two-year-old relies on parental support and encouragement, and on the security they engender, in order to develop a sense of his or her autonomy. It is precisely because a two-year-old knows that the parents are there that he or she can take the risks involved in beginning to move away from them.

Knowing that a loving, adult child will come to the rescue, if necessary, several of the elders in our study carry on with activities they have cherished for years, and maintain independent dwellings long after they might otherwise have stopped doing so. Some also rely on their children as a way to avoid the kind of anticipatory worry that leads many of their peers to restrict their activities. One widowed man says, in describing his current life, "I can stay up here in the woods because I know if I really need help, my son will be here inside of three hours. Now, this deal with fixing my own water pipes, I'd have never tried that without my son so near by, and I didn't even need him."

When their grown children have failed to provide necessary assistance, almost none of our informants speak blamingly. This omission may be related to the later-life reconciling of issues of generativity and stagnation, as was discussed in an earlier section. Although all of the elders in our study praise those forms of assistance that the children *do* provide, few bemoan those that are not forthcoming. Some make such excuses for their children as "She's so busy she can't be worrying about my doctors' appointments." Some speak of finding assistance elsewhere, for example: "For daily things, I wouldn't think of asking my sons to come all the way out here. I have other people I can call on."

To an extent, some of the elders in our study seem to feel they can maintain a sense of willful independence only in the presence of children who will provide a critical measure of protection against the consequences of behavioral deterioration. These individuals apparently cannot even admit that the children have failed them, and they go to great psychological lengths, if necessary, in order to avoid recognizing this failure and the helplessness it implies for them. One woman, whose children have been consistently inconsiderate and unreliable, both toward her and in their own lives, overtly denies this behavior. She asserts, "My daughter is so good to me. She treats me like a queen, like a piece of china. She is such a source of strength." This woman seems to be referring to herself when, later in the interview, she speaks sorrowfully of a poor neighbor who is perpetually victimized by her devilish, irresponsible offspring.

Caught between the wish to be self-sufficient and the recognition that they may need advice in some areas, our informants experience both security and stubbornness in response to their children's suggestions. This ambivalence contrasts with the grateful reliance on assistance, discussed above. Elders express a variety of views about the stubbornness of old people. The men espouse an exaggeration of the self-reliant stance that has characterized them throughout life. One asserts sweepingly, "I don't want any advice from anyone." He adds, "I don't want to have to blame anyone. I want to make up my own mind." Another admits, "You get kind of hardheaded when you get old. Even if you need it, you're not so ready to take advice from the young." Among the men, it seems that youth's fervent individualism and middle age's proud self-sufficiency tend to develop into old age's stubbornness, as themes of dependence and independence resurface throughout the life cycle.

Among women, this theme appears to take a rather different form. As we noted in earlier sections, the women in our study have demonstrated lifelong accommodation, reflected in the ways most of them have relied on their husbands, have subordinated their own dreams to those of other family members, and have nonetheless sought to retain a sense of self-determination. In old age, these women find themselves in a position of building on this foundation of accommodation, as they seek to take advantage of new opportunities for autonomous behavior. Although they share the men's tension between wishing to be independent and knowing that they must be able to rely on dependable others, they can often balance this tension more flexibly than their male counterparts. That is, they seem to be able to integrate stubbornness with diplomatic acquiescence far more comfortably than the men.

For example, a widow in her late eighties discusses her daughter's attempts to prevent her from eating foods that the doctor has forbidden. This woman prides herself on her ability to make her own decisions and, particularly since the death of her husband, to live on her own, in accord with her own wishes, interests, and capabilities. On the other hand, she is extremely proud of the daughters who have achieved both professional and marital success, thanks largely to our subject's ingenuity and devotion during those years when money was so scarce that she subordinated all other concerns to her efforts to keep the family fed and clothed. She is keenly aware that she has compromised her own immediate wishes throughout life, and that these compromises have had outcomes that she finds extremely gratifying. "When the children left," she says, "we were free to do as we pleased, without being limited by what was best for them. And since my husband died I have had no choice but to enjoy being free and being able to take care of myself. Now my daughter gets it into her head to start telling me what I shouldn't eat. Darned if I'm going to start taking orders again, at this point. It makes me so mad! But I just do it when she's not here. There's no point in provoking a fight when it can be avoided. There are some things you have to give in on a little bit."

As with the toddler absorbed in developing a sense of willfulness modified by appropriate doubt about his or her own capacities, so for the elder stubbornness and compliance may come to dominate psychosocial experience. One informant observes, "Stubbornness in old people is just self-defense. We know we need to listen," and that need apparently hurts. After all, many of these people have not *needed* to listen since they were children—when listening was a matter both of authority and of necessity. To them, old age's need to heed the warnings or instructions of others may represent a forced renunciation of adulthood, in much the same way we discussed earlier, with respect to giving up a license to drive. Some individuals reconcile this tendency toward compliance with an ongoing sense of autonomy by choosing specific experts to whose directives they will submit. For example, a man who has loved wine since his war years in Italy searched for a doctor who would permit him to drink wine, and he has adhered to all of that doctor's other dietary and behavioral restrictions. To other individuals, the sense of old-age autonomy simply cannot incorporate a compliance with newly imposed behavioral restrictions. These people may be gracious about demurring, but they remain intransigent. A diplomatically stubborn woman explains, "Everyone is so nice about what they think is good for me. If it's something I want to do my own way, I'm very stubborn, but I'm nice about it."

Stubbornness may be aroused between aged marital partners, particularly when one partner has primary responsibility for caring for a disabled spouse. Let us reconsider the couple discussed earlier, in connection with old-age intimacy and isolation as related to disability and caretaking. Remember that the disabled wife required so much care from her husband that they have recently moved into a small apartment in a facility that offers extensive medical services. In various ways, this man's own autonomy is threatened by his wife's deterioration. It is in order to accommodate her needs that he has had to move from a large home that he loved to a small apartment in a building populated with "old people who blow their noses at the dinner table and talk only about the weather." He offers her a steady barrage of advice, instructions, and restrictions, about which she is always passively stubborn. Afraid to leave her alone, he openly laments that he can go for a walk only when she has an hour with the physical therapist. But she is resentful of being palmed off so that he can get away from her, and she increasingly refuses to accept care or assistance from anyone except him. These two frequently find themselves locked in an unacknowledged contest of wills in which neither competitor can be either autonomous or victorious.

Among other elders, efforts to experience a sense of willful control may give rise to manipulative, intrusive behavior toward those with whom they interact. Some people who behave in this way may be reacting to perceived losses of personal autonomy by restricting the autonomy of others. For example, the woman in the couple just described is clearly manipulating her husband with her own helplessness. Manipulative behavior among our subjects most often appears to be largely unconscious, and it is frequently accompanied by one of the commonest assertions of the aging, "I don't want to inconvenience anyone; I don't want to be a burden, but . . ."

For other individuals, controlling or manipulative maneuvers seem to be a lifelong autonomy-related style rather than a new response to the circumstances and psychodynamics of later life. One woman, described in our historical data as perpetually overinvolved in and overcontrolling of her children's lives, may be viewed as exemplifying such old-age expression of a lifelong style. During our research interviews, she relentlessly controlled each session by telling long, over-detailed stories, each of which she introduced as tangential to the interviewer's last question. These stories proved to be uninterruptible, for when the interviewer broke in with a new question, the subject calmly continued her story from the point of interruption.

Many elders resent taking orders but are nonetheless willing to comply. For example, the wheelchair-bound woman discussed earlier, who now lives with her daughter, complains about having been rendered unnecessarily helpless when she was forbidden to clean or cook while she was living in a different daughter's home: "I couldn't have done much anyway, but those things were all I could do except sit like a lump, and she just wouldn't let me." Others, like the following woman, who now lives in a board-and-care home, quietly refuse to comply. "They even want to tell me what drawer to put my underwear in," she says. "So I just go along my own way and do things to suit myself." And some, like the following group of rural seniors that includes one of our informants, steer clear of restrictions altogether. During a recent windstorm, a large tree fell on and destroyed their center. After meeting with representatives of various governmental agencies, these people decided to build a new center for themselves, by themselves, rather than submit to any but the most basic of restrictions and regulations. A retired architect has designed a simple building. The group includes a number of retired carpenters, who are working at their own pace and are teaching some of the other elders. Where necessary, they are hiring outside labor to complete specific tasks. So that they will not have to stop meeting for the duration of the project, they have arranged for the midday use of a local church. Although their new center will not be completed for some time, it will be entirely *theirs,* and they are already enormously proud of it.

In an earlier chapter, we discussed various ways that individual attention to appearance and body image may be related to an old-age integration of lifelong identity and identity confusion. These concerns are also involved in the later-life struggle to balance a sense of strength and self-reliance with opposing feelings of shameful deterioration and resulting behavioral inadequacy. As they grapple with the inexorable process of growing old, many of our informants focus on one or another aspect of physical appearance. Some speak of learning to accept the clumsy and unsightly canes, hearing aids, bi- and trifocals, and wheelchairs that are now virtually body extensions. Others have struggled to accept the image of leaning on someone younger and stronger. One woman explains, "I've felt ashamed that it's hard to get up and walk, and to hold on to somebody's arm. But I don't feel ashamed any more. I'm grateful for it now." The acceptance of physical symbols of impairment without paralyzing shame has permitted these people to continue to express a goodly measure of autonomy.

By comparison, other elders are unable to accept devices they regard as graceless and ungainly, and they resolutely refuse to use them. It seems that shame at impairment has led these people to experience an unnecessarily disabling loss of autonomy. Two severely arthritic women mentioned earlier illustrate this stance. The first is ashamed at the thought of moving clumsily, without the elegance that has long been central to her self-image—and so she moves as little as possible. The second, doggedly self-reliant since childhood, cannot tolerate the feeling of helplessness she associates with using a wheelchair. She refuses to rely on any device more substantial than a cane, with the result that she cannot walk more than a few steps at a time, and then only within the supportive confines of her small apartment.

Some of our subjects, particularly the women, scrutinize

their faces each day in the mirror, experiencing a sense of satisfaction in characteristics of youthful appearance, and helplessness at inevitable characteristics of aging. One complains of the wrinkles, skin problems, and other disfigurements of old age, noting with wry pride that at least her hair stays naturally curly and doesn't turn gray. Some people describe the lifelong confidence and self-esteem inherent in their consistently young-looking appearances. One expresses her wish to be a blond ninety-year-old; others delight in the disbelief of strangers at being told their ages.

We believe that people in all stages of the life cycle may use personal appearance and grooming as a domain in which to act out conflicts between individual willfulness and social compliance. One woman in our study, in particular, appears to be engaged in just such a process. An avid reader of Hollywood news, she has long felt that given a fair opportunity, she, like the movie stars she admires, could rise above the circumstances that have always confined her. She maintains a costumed, doll-like appearance that flouts the dreariness of her surroundings and the colorlessness she perceives in the other tenants of her apartment building. She hosted her afternoon interviews wearing brocaded dresses and opulent jewelry, her face heavily powdered in a pale color and highlighted with vivid rouge and lipstick, in the style of a stage performer.

In far less unconventional ways, several other subjects are overly compliant or noncompliant with norms or opinions concerning appearance. One woman plays golf wearing the silk lounging pajamas and flowing chiffon scarves that give her the look of privileged femininity she has always cultivated. Another wears the brightly colored blouses her husband gets down from her closet for her, but occasionally she dons them inside out. A third appears increasingly dowdy, despite her avowed lifelong concern with good grooming as prescribed in women's magazines and newspaper fashion pages. All of these women express frustration with what they experience as the constriction and lack of freedom of their old age. Through her clothing, each seems to be proclaiming, publicly, that she is a person with a mind of her own, who is not willing to fade into oblivion.

By comparison, other women in our study use personal grooming as a vehicle for extreme acquiescence in, if not overcompliance with, societal convention. One such woman has long described herself primarily in terms of involvement with community organizations, social clubs, and groups of friends. In her youth she had been a swimmer, and in middle age she had resumed this activity for its physiological and recreational value. When she and her husband moved into a retirement community, she also took up golf and lawn bowling. In recent years, she has abandoned all of these forms of exercise, explaining, "I don't want to be seen in public with wet hair, and it's too tiring to swim with my head out of the water. And since my hernia, I don't look too pretty around the middle, here. It doesn't show much in a dress, but in golf clothes or a bowling outfit. . . . These little old ladies look silly, running around dressed like youngsters, and I don't want to be like that." This woman has always been accepted in whatever group she cared to join, and it is only recently that she finds herself beginning to worry about what people will think, rather than taking their approval and acceptance for granted. As she considers the possibility of social shame —a possibility that seems to be associated with a constricting environment, which necessarily increases the importance of any one element—she chooses to refrain from participating in various activities that she feels might diminish her social acceptability.

Whereas the elders just considered struggle to express willfulness by carefully attending to grooming, others among our informants seem to assert autonomy by demonstrating overall inattention to clothing and appearance. Although most of the people in this second group wear clothes that are clean and unwrinkled, and although many have money, have traveled, and have lovely objects displayed throughout their homes, they do not dress or groom in a way that indicates active concern with appearance. It is as if many of them are choosing not to waste time on an image they feel they cannot completely control—as if they believe that as long as they have not tried, and failed, to master the physical signs of aging, they can somehow escape the shame of losing control.

Physical safety in contemporary society is another issue related to our informants' sense of control over their own lives. Many mention safety as a concern that leads them deliberately to restrict their own behavior. Several will not go out at night, although they may feel lonely and bored. Some will not open their doors at all, unless a prospective caller has arranged a visit in advance. Many who continue to pursue some outside activity in the evenings make elaborate arrangements to travel only in groups, and even then they often find themselves so frightened that, when the next opportunity arises, they choose to stay home.

Some elders adapt to this perceived danger by going to bed almost immediately after dinner. Many watch more television than they think is good for them, as a way to fill evening hours they would prefer to be spending outside the home. Some have moved into retirement communities or into some form of residential facility primarily in order to be under the protection of elaborate security precautions. Nearly all of these people express the helpless feeling that they have no other choice. They may feel imprisoned by the night. They may feel cut off from friends, activities, and entertainment. They may regret that they must live in age-segregated communities. But they also believe that survival demands that they relinquish other alternatives. Only a few of our informants defiantly pursue whatever activities they choose, refusing to be restricted by a danger they believe should not exist in the first place. Even these few recognize that their behavior is risky and may be made riskier at any moment by a news report of a mugging, by a stiff back that impedes brisk walking, or by other uncontrollable occurrences.

Financial circumstances impose an additional influence on the control an individual is able to wield over his or her own life and the choices that determine its course. For the elderly, who are often on fixed incomes without apparent opportunities to supplement them, this influence is likely to be particularly restrictive. Appropriate housing and nutrition are critical, typically expensive conditions of the general health that is crucial to old-age self-reliance. Several of our informants find themselves relying on outside support to meet these basic needs. Those who cannot drive must have groceries brought in, if they are to maintain current levels of health and household independence. Those who cannot cook often depend on the Meals on Wheels program for the daily hot, balanced meal that is important to overall health.

Adequate medical care, often exceeding the services provided by Medicare, is essential if the elderly are to maintain behavioral autonomy in the face of inevitable physiological deteriorations. Potentially reversible conditions may lead to serious, irreversible disability or to death if they are not diagnosed correctly and treated promptly. Expensive rehabilitation care and compensatory services may also be necessary if the old person is to regain optimal independence after a disabling disease or accident. If a woman, living alone and recovering from a fall, for example, cannot afford to hire a housecleaner, she must either find a way to do minimally essential cleaning herself or live in a home that is increasingly dirty and uninhabitable.

Few of the people in our study talk openly or specifically about current finances. Two who are obviously wealthy acknowledge, "Financial security is really a terrific blessing when you're older. I can do what I like. I can hire whatever help I need. I will never go to a rest home." Many whose financial well-being is less secure matter-of-factly mention such bits of daily economy as being sparing with taxicabs, phoning the children on weekends or collect, and relying on the children's financial assistance in order to replace a well-maintained, old car that was destroyed while parked in a lot. It appears that for most of our informants, the ability to live adequately on the money at their disposal is an important part of a sense of independence in old age. They strive both to *demonstrate* autonomy on the basis of existing financial resources and to *experience* a sense of autonomy in whatever system of financial interdependence exists across family generations.

Our informants have lived their long lives in a society that extols the values of individuality, self-reliance, and independence. Throughout the life cycle, reexperiencing the theme of autonomy and shame/doubt has held a special societal meaning, alongside its integral psychosocial importance. In later life, as well, reconciling the syntonic and the dystonic elements of this theme is likely to invoke, in the individual, concerns about participation in and relationship to society as a whole. The elders in our study are proud of the extent to which they have lived as the willful, self-reliant individuals they were all taught to be, and they struggle valiantly to maintain this pride as the balance between self-determination and dependence shifts with the changing capacities of old age. One woman muses, "That's the worst thing. We want to keep doing, and we know we need help. But we have always learned to do everything on our own."

8. TRUST AND MISTRUST: HOPE

The tension between basic trust and mistrust reaches back to the very beginnings of life, when, through ever-growing trust in the reliable supportiveness and responsiveness of the environment, the healthy infant develops the origins of hope. This essential strength matures throughout the life cycle, as the individual struggles to integrate a sense of confidence and belief in the universe, and the relative predictability of its laws, with a discriminating cautiousness and skepticism about the same universe and its realistic unpredictabilities and unreliabilities. Throughout life, this tension involves issues of commitment to established religion and, with increasing age, of quasi-religious, philosophical considerations. Early concern with the predictability of the day-to-day world and immediate experience expands into concern with understanding the infinite universe in which all personal, practical knowledge is set. The strength of hopefulness that ideally comes to underlie the infant's earliest sensory awareness gradually becomes a basis for lifelong engagement with less directly knowable realms of experience. This basic initial strength sustains the healthy development of all subsequent psychosocial strengths. In old age, it is closely bound up with reinvolvement in all earlier psychosocial themes. At the end of life, we may find that some rudimentary hope has blossomed into a mature faith in being that is closely related to essential wisdom.

Grappling with current religious beliefs, and reconsidering the religious practices of a lifetime, our informants seek to reconcile opposing old-age tendencies toward trust and assurance, on the one hand, and toward wariness and uncertainty, on the other. Most of these people were raised in one or another of the formal Christian denominations. Many have remained in those same denominations, reciting the same prayers and raising their own children according to the same principles of faith that they learned as children. For them, religious involvement has been a source of continuity, throughout their own lives and across generations. And this very continuity has gradually become an object of faith, that is, something they feel they can count on, something in which they feel safe believing.

One woman reflects, "I learned a rhyming version of the Ten Commandments as a child, and I have never forgotten it. There are still some good things in there, if you stop to think about it." Although not necessarily consciously, this woman has, from childhood, lived her life according to the values inherent in these commandments. She has tried to make her own behavior conform to their instruction and to understand and respond to unexpected events in her family life in terms of their dicta. They have consistently provided her a reassuring foundation. Now, as she struggles to make sense of the life she has lived and the principles linking this individual life to something larger, those basic Judeo-Christian tenets from her earliest days emerge as an essential component of her belief system.

For some of the elders in our study, a reconciling of religious faith in old age must incorporate an earlier-life rejection of the religious training of childhood, in favor of an active, individual search for a more desirable religious doctrine. One woman describes having been raised in a devoutly

Lutheran family. Her father was the religious head of household, and his strict interpretation of the Bible and its commandments informed all religious instruction within the family. Our informant recalls, "My father was very loving and we all respected him, but his God was mean. I wanted to find a God of love." Paradoxically, the underlying beliefs she absorbed from her father's behavior seemed to conflict with the articulated principles that were part of his religious teachings. Throughout his professional life, her father had demonstrated a belief in resolute commitment to principle. He always disregarded community opinion in his dealings with individuals. As a merchant, he would sell to any client whose integrity he respected, regardless of that person's reputation in town. He always encouraged his children to rise above the petty teasing of their classmates, to ignore the superficial pain of jeers at unfashionable clothing and faded hair ribbons, and to draw strength from their own inner values. In matters of religion, however, he demonstrated a rigid intolerance that seemed to conflict with everything his daughter had learned from him about how to live daily life. When the time came for her to be confirmed in her father's religion, she respectfully declined.

She recalls, her expression first serious and then sparkling, "It nearly broke his heart. It was the first time one of us had overtly rejected something that was important to him. But I felt I was accepting everything he stood for, at the same time. He said I was breaking his heart. . . . He got over it." From the time of her adolescent rejection of unacceptable religious doctrine, this woman has devoted considerable lifelong effort to the exploration of a wide variety of religions, finally embracing what she describes as "a little religion that just teaches love." Her faith is by no means limited to the teachings of her adopted church. She uses these teachings simply as a scaffold around which she constructs an intricate, personal system of beliefs. For her, choosing a particular denomination had to do with finding an ideology, a view of God and the universe, that was not incompatible with the convictions she was continuing to develop within herself, as a result of a thoughtful consideration of her life, her teachers, and her studies. Reconciling her feelings of belief and disbelief in old age involves continuing her lifelong practice of thoughtful reconsideration, diligent study, and commitment to basic principles.

The majority of our informants demonstrate some level of active concern with understanding humankind's place in the universe. Some of these people now attend church more regularly than they have in years. As they find their thoughts focusing on issues of faith, so they seem to find their lives centering on church-based services and activities. Their congregations tend to be small and interdenominational, having, at least superficially, little to do with the denominational formalities that they observed in earlier years. Whereas subtle theological commitments may have been important in the middle-age churchgoing of these people, attendance in old age seems to be prompted by less differentiated needs simply to participate in religion and to affirm a basic faith.

Other informants seem to satisfy these same undifferentiated needs without physically attending church. Some of these people are able to experience religious faith by listening to church services on the television or radio. A woman explains, "I'm afraid I can't get to church as often as I should. But I listen on the radio every Sunday morning. Three or four different churches on the radio. I'm as close to God here as anywhere else." Others renew a sense of faithfulness by praying alone, without the structure of a formal service of any kind. One woman reasons, "Prayer is being in accord with the Deity. Good is the basis of everything, and mishap is getting out of touch, out of step, out of harmony." To this woman and others like her, it is individual praying rather than formal theology or structured group worship that is at the heart of the later-life reintegration of trust and mistrust through religious faith.

Many elders puzzle over the relation between organized religion and human life, concluding that since the "whole idea of religion is to build better people, . . . to make a better world, then basic moral values" are, in fact, the essence of religion. These people endeavor to articulate just what it is that they mean when they affirm belief in a personal God, a higher being, or a grand plan. Their individual meanings vary widely, emerging, as they do, from unique lifetimes of experience. However, each of these highly personalized meanings is rooted in a struggle that transcends individual informants. That is, each elder is seeking to balance a lifelong sense of security with an opposing lifelong sense of insecurity, as part of an effort to place his or her own life in the context of a world that is larger than they have been able to see, that existed before they were born, and that will continue to exist after they have died.

One man avows his belief in a sense of immanent justice, a conviction that when everything is sorted out, those who have lived at the expense of others will get what is coming to them. This man, the writer of advertising jingles and slogans whom we discussed in earlier chapters, has long felt that life has not been fair to him. Although he was a master at his craft, outstanding success always seemed to pass him by, in favor of his competitors who were less than scrupulous about issues of plagiarism and unspoken agreements. For years, he railed against the conscience that forced him to practice human decency in an arena in which cutthroat op-

portunism was essential to highest achievement. He continues to grapple with these issues in old age, trying to reconcile
perceived professional failure with experienced moral success, in a way that does not force him to conclude either that
the world is inherently unfair or that his belief in the Golden
Rule is misplaced. His faith in immanent justice appears to
be such a reconciliation.

One of the oldest men in our study understands his extreme longevity as part of God's grand, inaccessible plan.
Raised as a devout Catholic, this man was orphaned young,
was denied the opportunity for prolonged education, and
was seriously injured several times before middle adulthood.
He drifted away from the church as he moved from one
community to another, trying to recover from each setback
and to establish a stable life course. He never rejected the
importance of religion in daily life, but the continually harsh
circumstances of his own life led him to abandon his childhood conviction that getting down on his knees and praying
to God would keep him well. "I did a lot of praying on these
knees," he says, "and I kept getting hurt anyway." He uses
bitter humor as one way to accept his disappointment in the
God of his childhood. "I'm not so egotistical as to think that
God is [made] after *our* image. It makes me laugh that
people would think that God is like us." Now in his late
nineties, this man has outlived his wife, his professional use-
fulness, his friends, his physical strength, and his zest. Particularly in these recent, weary years, he has struggled to reconcile empirical disillusionment with a need to believe, finally
resolving this lifelong tension by coming to a faith in the
inscrutability of God's grand plan. "There must be some
reason for you to live so long," he asserts. "Otherwise you
wouldn't [still] be living. I really believe that. . . . You come
onto the earth and you go through a lifetime and it really

isn't a long time, compared to the world and everything in it. We are almost a dot, and why we are here I really don't know. I have always regarded life as a mystery that way. . . . It's all part of a grand plan that God has for the world. But He is not accessible to individual people."

These individualized systems of belief represent personal expressions of confidence and security in some entity or order outside the self. The very specificity of these expressions, however, indicates that each is the product of a sincere personal struggle to trust in the face of mistrust, to accept in the face of the incomprehensible. The way in which these informants, and others, deny adherence to any one organized religion suggests the integration of a measure of thoughtful mistrust. They struggle to articulate criticism of the church, without renouncing an underlying sense of faith. One observes wryly, "The church isn't living up to the Father's good politics." This woman feels that she can practice these "good politics" on her own far more effectively than she could as part of a corrupted organization. Some of these people directly criticize or question their God for permitting innocent people to suffer. They waver about maintaining faith in such a questionable deity, but achieve a satisfactory resolution by asserting their conviction that faith must be stronger than human logic. Like the man in his nineties mentioned above, several comfort themselves with the thoughts that "we can't know His ways" and that "we are not supposed to understand."

One woman reasons, "There must be a God. Else how could all of these things be—people and trees and flowers? If I thought there wasn't a God, I'd have to go out and do something myself about all the bad people." Historical data suggest that this woman has long complained about the ways social and economic inequities have adversely affected her

family. However, although her criticisms were community-
and societywide in scope, she has always occupied herself
almost entirely with her family. Although she makes astute
observations about societal organization, she has never tried
to act on these observations by such means as attending
community meetings, writing to elected officials, or submit-
ting letters to a newspaper editor. This woman's trust in
herself and her own responsibilities in the world is intertwined with her trust in a God. If she can believe in a God,
she is free to question the way the world works, while leaving
the important action to God. She seems to feel that if there
were no God, however, she would have no choice but to act
on, rather than merely to reflect on or talk about, what she
believes to be right.

For several of our informants, efforts to integrate feelings
of security with those of misgiving have led to an abiding
faith in nature. One muses, "When I'm out in the open and
look up at the sky or at the stars, I have a feeling of closeness
with the stars." Another asks, "Have you ever been on the
top of a mountain and looked out, and the world is all there
and you feel, 'Gee, this is a darned good world after all'? That
restores my faith faster than anything else." A third asserts,
"All the serenity of nature is a symbol for me of immortality." For these individuals, faith as it emerges in in old age
is clearly affected by lifelong involvement with the natural
environment that often profoundly influences people who
have lived close to the land. One took refuge in the midwest-
ern woods as a child, and became a grower in California's
fertile Central Valley as an adult. The second grew up in a
rural mountain town, and has remained a devoted hiker and
backpacker to this day. The third lived, until recently, on a
large estate that included formal gardens and vineyards as
well as undeveloped wilderness that the surrounding com-

munity protected as a wildlife preserve. Regardless of religious affiliation, these individuals all demonstrate a deep sense that they and their lives are but one part of a world that has comprised everything we recognize as life and that will continue to do so as long as life continues to exist.

Most of our subjects seem convinced that it is important for their children and grandchildren to go to church—in order "to get values," "to be in harmony," or "to have something to lean on" or simply because "it's important." Those whose progeny do not attend church express disappointment, criticism, and resignation. Only one woman is able to understand this departure from her own belief system as acceptable, explaining, "Maybe the grandchildren are not old enough yet to need God very badly." If advanced age, in and of itself, is a criterion for needing God, our subjects are certainly old enough. Perhaps this is why they struggle so hard to define a God in whom they can believe, despite their very realistic doubts and criticisms.

It is interesting to note that many of our informants' expressed wishes for the younger generations to attend religious services bear little relation to their own attendance. As we discussed above, these elders demonstrate widely disparate forms of religious behavior, and they have highly individualized reasons for the nature of their current association, or lack thereof, with formal religion. Nevertheless, even many of those who have not attended a religious service in years say it is important for the next generations to do so now. They cannot explain this discrepancy, and we are left to speculate about its meaning. It seems that our informants view regular church attendance as a kind of ideal—a wholesome, rewarding expression of the kind of wholehearted faith they wish they could share. In these terms, they may view their own relative dissociation as the product of a lifelong struggle to come to terms with issues of faith. Even though the product of this struggle may depart from the ideal, the elders must honor it in order to maintain a sense of integrity. But they view the children and grandchildren as another matter.

Perhaps they think that the younger generations have not had time to engage in enough soul-searching to be justified in abandoning the ideal so early in life. Perhaps they feel that attending church provides the individual a kind of protection against painful uncertainty and mistrust, and they want the next generations to be protected. Perhaps, from the vantage point of old age, they feel that only after an early and middle life of relatively unquestioning participation in formal religion can personal feelings of faith be deeply enough ingrained to survive the kind of newly serious questioning that emerges as part of later life. Perhaps, too, their own, individualized belief systems include an unspoken, even unacknowledged, conviction that "going to church," and the complex of values and commitments this phrase represents, may somehow provide for their progeny a protection against the very real physical and emotional dangers of living in today's world. As grandparents, they have admitted that they do not know how to offer the protection they so desperately want the next generations to have. Perhaps coming to terms with personal mistrust has given them a faith that, through the reciprocal covenants of formal religion, God will protect their offspring in a way that they themselves are not able to do.

Many of our informants describe renewed religious activity around the death of a loved one—a spouse, a child, or a sibling. They are unable to explain their reasons for "returning to the fold," any more than to say, "I felt it was something I needed." Whatever the individual dynamics, this paradigm of religious reawakening at the loss of a loved one suggests that elders somehow struggle to deal with life's most profound, keenly felt unpredictabilities by believing in something that can transcend the present moment. That is, they tolerate deeply troubling skepticism and unpredictability by struggling to believe in something that promises security.

A number of our subjects put this dynamic into words as they conclude that the end of the world is coming, exactly as the Bible predicts. One explains, "Right now I think that the end of the world is coming. The Bible says that all nations shall be at war with each other, and we are so close to that now, aren't we?" A second asserts, "Things are in their last days. [It is written that] all these things are to happen in the last days." Terrified by the potential for a destruction so massive as to be unthinkable, these people succeed in tolerating their personal fear by recasting it as an already prophesied part of a trusted master plan.

As epigenetic theory explains, an early-developed sense of hope underlies the individual's subsequent integration of autonomy with shame/doubt, of initiative with guilt, of industry with inferiority, and so forth, throughout the life cycle. Thus, the capacity to be trustful in the face of realistic mistrust remains closely intertwined with all other psychosocial themes, and in old age it plays an important part in the way the individual reexperiences the psychosocial tensions of a lifetime. For example, confidence in the environment and reliance on one's own body are integral to various aspects of the later-life struggle for independence, discussed earlier as key to balancing the tension between autonomy and shame/doubt.

In an earlier section, we discussed ways that living in a long-familier home or neighborhood can support both an elder's internal feelings of willful self-determination and his or her realistically independent behavior. In addition to this contribution to autonomy in old age, having lived in the same house or neighborhood for more than thirty years seems to provide many of our informants feelings of stability and predictability that are closely linked with trustfulness throughout the life cycle. This issue of residential continuity as a source of supportive rootedness may be a new one, in our current age of geographic mobility. In an historical era in which people were likely to be born, to live, and to die in the same small village, such stability could be counted on. Today this sense of continuity is far more uncertain, noteworthy where it exists rather than where it does not. Our group of elders is somewhat unusual in this regard, in that we deliberately chose from our potential informants those individuals who live no more than a four-hour drive from Berkeley—the town in which they lived fifty-five years ago. In fact, some of these individuals still live in homes they have occupied for well over fifty years. By definition, then, many of our subjects have chosen to maximize this aspect of stability and predictability.

Money is another autonomy-related issue in connection with which the aged must integrate their sense of trust in a secure future with concern and doubtfulness about adequate support. This connection between money and basic security is lifelong. Although current recollections may bear relatively little relation to historical data on family financial circumstances, several of our informants report decades and more of anxiety about whether there would be enough money to make it through the month, to cover an emergency that might arise, to support retirement—in short, whether there would be enough money to ensure a future. These people invariably recall happiness in earlier life as coinciding with periods of financial security and prosperity. For them, financial ill- or well-being has long determined the feelings of hopefulness about the future that have always competed with feelings of uncertainty. The man who made a living by writing advertising slogans and jingles is such a person. When he talks about times when his income was good, he speaks with optimism about his own long-range goals and the future successes he anticipates for his children. However, when he describes times when his income was low, his time frame shifts from the long to the very short range, and his tone shifts from optimistic to doubtful and pessimistic. As he discusses his earlier life, he relaxes perceptibly when he begins to talk about the money he earned in the decade before retirement—money that has secured old age for him and his wife. It is not that he is unambivalent about his work during this decade or that he is wholly satisfied with the life he and his wife are sharing today, as earlier references to this couple suggest. Rather, it is that dissatisfaction in these later periods of financial security does not seem to carry the deep-seated, extremely unsettling sense of mistrust in a hostile environment that characterizes his expressed dissatisfaction with periods of monetary chanciness.

This psychological importance of financial security to some individuals is highlighted by its contrast with comments from others of our informants, whose lifelong financial circumstances have also been tenuous but who recall past instances of reassuring generosity and support, rather than those of fearful uncertainty. For example, in describing family circumstances during the Depression, one woman emphasizes that although they were desperately poor, "everyone was at the same level, and people were so good to one another." Rather than dwell on the lost jobs and frighteningly insecure finances that plagued her family, this woman chooses to discuss the assistance that was warmly offered by friends and relatives; she paints a vivid image of a check that arrived just in time for her and her husband to provide a Christmas celebration for their two small children. It is striking that this second group of elders seems to consider the present and future more in terms of things to do and people to love than of financial resources.

In only two of our subjects do we note a pervasive sense of current financial precariousness, and in both of them this sense seems to be related to serious doubtfulness and apprehension about the future. Most of our informants enjoy both a measure of personal financial security and a realistic reliance on financial security in the next generation, so that they may be relatively confident of being well taken care of as they continue to age. These two individuals, in contrast, are among the poorest in our sample, and their children seem to be either financially insecure, too, or unwilling to demonstrate any responsibility for their parents' well-being. Money intrudes often into their thoughts and conversation. They find themselves speaking of having been deprived and shortchanged, or overtly swindled and misled, in response to questions concerning such diverse life arenas as schooling, marriage, working, and child rearing. They introduce issues of costliness into discussions of favorite books, friends, and recreation.

When they talk of a future as immediate as tomorrow or next week, they invariably invoke a measure of uncertainty with qualifications like "I don't know what will happen, but . . ." or "If my friend still wants to, we might. . . ." In early life, both of these individuals seem to have been deprived of a good deal of the unconditional support and acceptance that characterizes the experience of most loved, healthy infants. In middle life, as well, they seem to have had to endure considerable uncertainty in regard to both financial and interpersonal circumstances. In later life, it seems that they cannot place realistic trust in friends, family, or finances. Their incessant references to monetary apprehension, deprivation, and capriciousness may well represent the only terms in which they are able to give voice to terrifying doubts about the hand they will be dealt, in a future that feels as unpredictable as a card game.

Physical health and ill health represent additional autonomy-related concerns around which our informants struggle to master anxieties that challenge their basic sense of certainty and security in the world. They know that their bodies are deteriorating, that they cannot be counted on to perform as they once did. Nonetheless, these elders are challenged to integrate appropriate mistrust of their own strength and of such rudimentary physical capacities as walking with a steadfast belief in their own physical survivability. One woman who nearly died as a young mother speaks glowingly of the doctor who saved her and refused the payment she could not have afforded. Her sense of confidence has always been high, and it is not surprising that she interprets current physical deterioration and earlier-life illness in terms of this underlying faith in a world that is supportive of her will to endure.

Another woman, now in her nineties, who was not expected to survive any of several critical childhood illnesses, speaks with contempt and suspicion of all doctors, to this very day. She has a fighter's wary confidence in her body's ability to survive whatever adversity an inhospitable, untrustworthy world is likely to offer. Notably, few, if any, of the elders in our study directly indicate a lack of trust in their own capacities, when speaking to us of their health. It seems, instead, that they are inclined to redirect a blaming mistrust and suspicion toward their physicians and toward lawyers, clergy, and other authorities on whom they must rely.

Diminished energy and sensory acuity, and resulting doubts about bodily reliability, may also be related to the later-life tension between initiative and guilt. Throughout life, the senses represent our primary basis for interacting with the world. From earliest life, the infant must come to trust his or her senses as a source of information about the environment. In childhood, sensory perception becomes the foundation for the playfulness and exploration that give rise to lifelong purposeful activity. It is not simply that diminished physical capacities challenge the elder's feelings of ingenuity and enthusiasm for activity, as we discussed earlier. In addition, these diminutions threaten the older person's sense of a predictable, knowable world as mediated by the senses and experienced through activity. Consider the woman, mentioned earlier, who complains of missing the symphony but who does not listen to the orchestral records provided by her son. Physical incapacitations make it impossible for her to attend concerts, as she has long enjoyed doing. In addition, we may speculate that these same incapacitations, and perhaps a touch of hearing loss, diminish her enjoyment of the music itself. If so, this lifelong music lover suddenly finds herself unable to count on music as her major source of pleasure. Alongside a later-life psychosocial imbalance in regard to participating in activity, she also confronts a sudden unpredictability in that particular mode of interaction with the world in which she has trusted, far more deeply than she can put into words.

Several of our informants express a basic, lifelong faith in the virtue and strength-giving properties of hard, disciplined, productive work. Some of these refer to working in terms of career; others, in terms of making a living. Still others seem to view as their most important work the transmission of their own values to the next generations. Regardless of the focus of their efforts, all of these people seem to have a near-religious faith in industriousness and competence. The orchard growers discussed in an earlier section exemplify this belief. Almost as other people insist that trusting in God and living according to the Ten Commandments are the bases for personal well-being in the world, these people have always been convinced that working hard is the only reliable source of strength. They look back on times of family crisis, and they point to the productive working that enabled them to endure. In old age, they continue to work in the orchards, even though they have handed down administrative responsibilities to their children. As a later-life foray into recreation, the husband in this couple now spends some time on theoretical research related to the cultivation of the fruits and nuts to which he has devoted so much vocational energy over the years. For these people, it is not only a renewed sense of competence that emerges from later life's integration of enterprise and effort, on the one hand, and laziness and halfheartedness, on the other. For them, this integration is inextricably intertwined with the renewal of their faith in something no less basic than a secure role in the world.

The tension between identity and identity confusion is tied to a sense of abiding faith, perhaps more closely than is any other psychosocial theme in old age. The concern with existential identity, described earlier, with reaffirming commitments that best reflect the "I" in the totality of life—such a concern is inseparable from the efforts, discussed at the outset of this section, to participate in a belief system that clarifies the individual's place in an infinite and timeless universe. In old age's reintegration of a sense of "I" as distinct from all of that which is not "I," religion may come to represent the "ultimate other." As living, personal heroes die away, elders may come to find themselves looking up to the immortal heroes of religion and to the timeless, infinitely trustworthy qualities they represent. Renewing a later-life balance between feelings of identity and those of identity confusion involves the individual in an effort to come to terms with the unique complex of beliefs and commitments faithfully held that constitutes a lifelong sense of self. The enduring beliefs that make up identity provide an important element of consistency and predictability over time. Also, they are part of the process through which the elder seeks to have faith in him- or herself over a lifetime, as part of a world that is inscrutable.

For many of our informants, various aspects of intimacy contribute to a sense of trustfulness in old age. Several people describe the church not only as a site for the expression of religious faith but also, perhaps even more important, as the center of their social lives. For some, this social focus is an expectable outgrowth of earlier-life involvement. In his younger years, one man assisted with the construction work on a new, community church building. A woman recalls her efforts to raise building funds for the local church in which she hoped to rear her children. In old age, some of these people help with church gardening and other light maintenance work, as a way to remain active and productive members of a community in which they have faithfully participated for decades. These elders and others like them have found their friends among church members, and their activities have been based in the church. They have relied on the church as a source both of religious commitment and of interpersonal security. Today the church continues to provide dependable security in these two realms. In highly individualized ways, it remains the basis for spiritual belief. More prominent in the day-to-day lives of our informants,

however, it also remains the basis for consistent social con-
nectedness. Once these people engaged in community out-
reach activities. Now they feel secure relying on regular
telephone calls from concerned church members, who seek
to make sure that these community elders are surviving from
day to day and that they know their involvement continues
to be valued.

For other people, the church and the hope it supports are
differently related to intimacy. For them, the church and its
clergy and congregation are a source of essential understanding, on the basis of which faith may be experienced as part
of an unconditional love and acceptance. One often cantan-
kerous man continues to attend Unitarian fellowship every
Sunday, as he has since childhood. Although he is sad frequently to find himself quarreling with neighbors and family
about issues of social policy and political movements, he feels
reassured that other church members understand his basic
commitments. He explains, "Unitarians have very strong
feelings about matters of social conscience and human concern. I trust their views, and they respect my principles. So
we won't walk off in a huff or be contemptuous of one another." After at least fifty years, a recently widowed woman
has resumed the practice of Catholicism. Reassurance in the
faith of her childhood is certainly one reason for her resump-
tion. Another important one is a search for the concern and
acceptance of intimacy, in the face of the loss of a lifelong
partner to whom she directed a near-spiritual devotion. She
muses, "I am looking for a priest who will listen to me as he
always listened—who will understand my life and accept
me."

Linking hope with generativity, many of our informants
express an ultimate faith in family and the generational cycle.
By and large, these are people who have deeply committed

themselves to family relationships throughout life and who have derived considerable satisfaction and a sense of self from acting on these commitments. As young parents, some involved the children in their own vocational and avocational activities. Others built their own lives around what they felt were the best interests of their children or, for periods, their aged parents. Some of these people describe a lifelong, absolute belief in their parents and/or grandparents, both as dependable caretakers and as implicitly trustworthy models for living life—as Elders. Most avow an unquestioning trust in their children today. Although they may disagree with various of the children's choices or actions, they differentiate this disagreement from their underlying, unqualified faith in the children as custodians of the world. One man concludes, "The hope of the world is in the younger generations." These elders hold a comforting, absolute faith in the family, as an anchor in a world that is often tempestuous. They experience "a feeling of security about family": "You don't worry about it. You just know that that is your family and that they are all with you."

Among our elders' comments are those that reflect exaggerated extremes of trustfulness and mistrustfulness. The first extreme is illustrated by those who assert, in absolute tones that permit no doubt, that they will be taken care of, no matter what—even though instances of need have arisen and the expected caretakers have failed to provide. As with various aspects of faith in a God, as we discussed earlier, these elders seem to need to trust in the sense of responsibility of others, even when such trust demands that they ignore a realistic cause for a measure of doubt. The opposite extreme is illustrated by those for whom the primary mode of experiencing the world seems to be one of blaming, of mistrusting, and of criticizing people and circumstances. For these people, any activity seems to represent an opportunity to display apprehension; any encounter becomes an occasion to recall past affronts and injustices. Somewhere between these two extremes lies the expression of mature faith. Evolving from lifelong experiences of hopeful confidence and cautious skepticism, faith that is sturdy and firm need not itself be questioned. As one woman declares, "Faith is one of those things. You don't bother to go into it too much. It just *is.*"

III

A Life History:
Revisitation
and Reinvolvement

I. THE SCREENPLAY

The choice of a screen personality as a truly meaningful model of a human life calls for an explanation. The fact is that this film was regularly used near the finale of a Harvard course called "The Human Life Cycle," because of the totally convincing way in which it presents an old man's survey —in memories, fantasies, and dreams—of the stages and the places of his development as a child, a man, and a doctor. And since then we have come to prefer this moving picture to any other life history or case history at our disposal, for it illuminates them all while ever again adding most artful credence to the assumption of some vital involvements typical for what we believe to be universally given stages of life. All this seems to be deeply understood by Ingmar Bergman.* But we know that in briefly describing his work, which obvi-

---

*See EHE's previous descriptions of *Wild Strawberries* in Erik H. Erikson, ed., *Adulthood* (New York: W. W. Norton, 1978), 1–24.

ously needs to be seen and heard, we make the reader take a double chance: with our review of the motion picture as well as with the "fictitious" life offered in it. Yet, we would claim that students faced with any story of a life as presented in more "scientific" media, such as case histories or statistical summaries, are confronted with no less of a combination of freedom and constriction on the part of their reporters. Of these, we have mentioned the necessity to guard their subject's privacy, while attempting to prove as logical and trustworthy their method of selecting their "data."* All this, taken together, may well make, on occasion, for more distortion than clarification. And when we consider a research study of the kind described in this book as consisting of the life data entrusted to academic investigators, mostly in interviews, by the surviving members of a representative group of parents in Berkeley, California, it must be obvious how cautious we have to be in our publication, especially in describing often highly confidential details we ourselves have every reason to consider to be among the most vital or dynamic experiences in those lives. But there is also a more positive reason for the choice of a work of art for our purposes. Our own approach forces us, from the outset, to keep in mind the question of what determines the overall coherence, the "gestalt," of a whole life. Here we may well take into account the larger fact that artistic works of greatness have a way of presenting in a convincing form some total truths about life, which rarely characterize other reports and abstracts of a human life, making it truly a life history—within the generational process.

---

*We have recently seen a document to be signed by the contributors to a psychoanalytical publication in which they are expected to promise (no doubt, on good legal grounds) that all case material has been sufficiently disguised to be unrecognizable—even to the patient.

Here we may point out, too, that our great teacher Sigmund Freud named one of his most salient observations in daily clinical work the Oedipus complex, which describes the fate of a son figure in a classical drama. (This proved revolutionary, even if today some of us would not wish to let the father, Laius, get away so easily with blaming his own actions entirely on his little son's threatening intentions, which the oracle had prophesied.)

To summarize, we believe that we can best begin to demonstrate more pictorially some of the dynamics of the interwoven stages of human life, as they culminate in old age, by outlining the scenes and the themes that reveal, in Bergman's drama, an old man's search for his life's transcendent meaning; and by claiming that all old people are involved in some such search, whether they—or we—know it or not.

It is, then, important and very helpful for our purposes that Dr. Borg's story begins with a time in his life when something seems to have made him acutely curious regarding themes in his life. We thus first see him at the age of seventy-six sitting at his (most orderly) desk in his suburban apartment in Sweden, starting a journal of a sequence of events he had just lived through. The first "event," of all things, is a frightening dream he had in the night preceding this special day, on which he was planning to travel to the university town of Lund to receive, at a "Jubilee" ceremony, the highest Swedish award for a physician: an honorary degree crowning him with a famous black cylinder for having been a doctor for fifty years. It is a sober man who now, on returning from that trip, reconstructs for himself one after the other his state of mind when awakening from that dream; his leaving for Lund, and a series of astonishing experiences, and dreams, on the way there; and the great ceremony itself. At the end, we will see whether what "moved" him on that day to such a special sense of self-awareness was only the expectation of the great honor that was awaiting him with all the ritual symbols of a professional superidentity, or whether there was somebody or something that forced him to recognize in himself some decisive lack of vital involvement in his old age.

Dr. Isak Borg, as we first hear him identify himself, is a retired Swedish doctor and, of course, a Lutheran: a *mighty fortress* in Swedish is a *vaeldig borg.* He is the only one left of ten brothers and sisters—a rare survivor, then, as was once typical for the oldest individuals alive, and a high-class "elder" rather than one of numerous "elderlies" of today. His very first sentence, it so happens, lands us in the middle of one of the terminological quandaries to be dealt with in this book, for we assign to the dominant (psychosocial) tension of the last stage of life a certain syntonic sense of integrity, as well as a dystonic one of despair. And the doctor's first sentence is "At the age of seventy-six, I feel that I'm much too old to lie to myself."* There follows a *but*—"But of course I can't be too sure"—and a cautious rationalization of his self-isolation or (in terms of our study) his disinvolvement. All he asks of life is "to be left alone and to have the opportunity to devote [him]self to the few things which continue to interest [him]." Here he mentions golf, detective stories, and the latest developments in his "beloved" science: bacteriology. This is the only use of the word *beloved.*

As to his family, he has a son in Lund, also a doctor, who has no children. His mother is ninety-six; she and he seldom see each other. His (now all dead) brothers and sisters left some children and grandchildren, with whom he has "very

---

*This and subsequent quotations are taken from *Four Screenplays of Ingmar Bergman,* trans. Lars Malmstrom and David Kushner (New York: Simon and Schuster, 1960).

little contact." His wife is dead: the marriage was "quite unhappy." As for his present company, he refers only to his "good housekeeper," an old woman. Finally, he calls himself an "old pedant" who detests emotional outbursts, women's tears, and the crying of children. All of these simple themes will become significant as we proceed. He, at this point, tells of a dream that "befell him"—a nightmare, in fact, and apparently one of a whole series in recent years.

Dr. Borg's dreams, of course, "must be seen." But so must all the events. We can underline only some themes that point to this old man's deep, if not altogether conscious, old-age despair.

The Nightmare

One early summer morning (and in Sweden this can mean 2 A.M.), Dr. Borg dreams that he is taking his regular morning stroll in streets unusually empty for a weekday. Even on the sunny side, it is chilly, and his footsteps echo in an absolute silence. The big clock over the door of the watchmaker-optometrist has no hands, and when he holds his own watch to his ear, he hears his own heart beat. On turning back toward home, he "to his joy" sees someone, but it is a man who proves to have "no face" (it actually is a face with tightly closed eyes and mouth) and who at that moment collapses and then disappears into the pile of clothes on the street.

The dreamer now finds himself in a strange part of the city. An approaching hearse begins to sway and rock, like a baby's cradle—and, indeed, makes a noise reminiscent of a baby's cry. Finally, a coffin is thrown out on the street, and as he peers into it with fearful curiosity, he sees a corpse inside, which looks like himself and (with a "scornful smile") grabs

his arm: this wakes him up. One is left with a rich symbolism
of life and death—even his own corpse, trying to lure him
toward his certain fate, and, close to it, the most delicate cry
of a newborn baby.

The Decision

Awakening from all this "senseless horror," Dr. Borg
makes a decision that will immediately bring him into confrontation with Agda, his only slightly younger housekeeper
(for forty years). We learn of his decision as he confronts her
with it, not without arousing some conversational themes
illustrating what in our work we call the "disdain" (and only
too obvious) "self-disdain" of old people. When he hurriedly
enters her bedroom, apparently not quite covered up by his
dressing gown, she sits up and asks, "Are you ill, Professor?"
When told of his decision to travel to Lund by car instead
of by air, as had carefully been planned, she complains that
he is ruining "the most solemn day" of her life, and in the
exchange that follows he eventually says, "We are not married," to which she responds, "I thank God every night that
we're not"—decades of bickering condensed in minutes.

Bergman's genius now has sketched the daily circumstances of Dr. Borg's old age, all contained in an isolation
that is about to be gloriously interrupted (but possibly only
interrupted) by his drive to the crowning ceremony in the
cathedral at Lund. In the next moment, however, a new
person appears. As Agda pointedly turns her back on Dr.
Borg and his coffee, a door opens and a beautiful young
woman (wearing pajamas and smoking a cigarette) appears:
it is Marianne, the wife of Dr. Borg's son, Evald. (She apparently has been staying for some weeks with the doctor and
Agda without any full explanation for her being away from

home.) She must have heard, through the walls, of his plan to go to Lund by car: "May I go with you? . . . I want to go home." "Home?" Isak asks pointedly. "Home to Evald?" But he agrees, and she withdraws again, to get ready.

We cannot at this point help asking ourselves what stage of life this Marianne must be representing. All we know about her so far is that she is childless. Yet, her age suggests that her stage of life, and Evald's, is that of generativity versus stagnation, which provides the psychosocial dynamics for a strong wish to take care.

The Departure

But now we have the privilege of seeing this couple drive through an early Swedish summer morning around a suburban circle and into the country. And we witness Bergman's mastery in making of an automobile a moving stage for human confrontation.

It begins, in all that beauty of the passing landscape, with some leftovers of a rather disdainful emotionality that is hard to take from such a handsome couple of mature faces seen next to each other in the front seats of a car "conversing" without being able to confront each other directly. But obviously, also, both conversants feel a need to be honest with each other.

It all begins with the petty issue of whether she may smoke a cigarette, and this leads him to talk disdainfully of women smokers. She tries to shift to the topic of the weather; on that, they agree, there *will* be a storm, indeed. She asks for his "real age"; he claims to know what she is thinking of, namely, some money Evald owes his old father. He insists that Evald knows he owes it to him, for his son and he share some principles; and now she lets him have it: yes, but Evald hates him, too. Isak, for a moment, looks thunderstruck. But she now confesses that she had a month earlier come to ask him for help and that in reply he had used some truly nasty phrases, such as "suffering of the soul," "spiritual masturbation," and "quacks and ministers." Finally, they both laugh somewhat relaxedly—and, unbelievably, he says he wants to tell her a dream—the dream, no doubt, just reported. But she claims to have no interest in dreams. All such talk, then, seems to reflect some typical trends in the feeling of old and middle-aged individuals as they are testing out some more or less healthy disdain and rejectivity, and yet also to reveal their need for each other as fatherly and motherly friends, respectively. But why now, and on that trip? This we have yet to learn. In the meantime, we can only conclude that Marianne seems eager to confront him with his obsessive involvements and with his lack of vital ones. (But what, indeed, is she so deeply involved in herself?)

The Strawberry Patch

Isak suddenly (or so he says) decides to turn into a small side road, down to the sea. This he does "by impulse," he claims even in his journal, but it will be clear presently that that little "side road" leads to one of the scenes to be revisited and which prompted him to take the car in the first place.

Driving down that winding road, Isak repeats his offer to share things with her: he wants to "show her something." But she sighs quietly, and as a large old yellow summerhouse comes into sight among birch trees she declares its style to be a bit ridiculous and excuses herself: she wants to "take a dip." Isak explains that this is the house in which his family spent the summers of his first twenty years; and he begins to have a "strange feeling of solemnity." In fact, he is looking for a particular spot he had wanted to show her—yes, a patch of wild strawberries! He finds it and, now alone, sits down to eat some berries slowly, as if they contained some consciousness-expanding essence. And indeed, the real scene and dreamlike images now begin to fuse, and the old mind's involvement in memories comes out in scenes that a motion picture can convey especially well. He suddenly "sees" *her:* Sara, his erstwhile sweetheart, a "lighthearted young blonde" in a "sun-yellow dress" gathering strawberries. She is so close he could touch her—if he dared. And then, he sees his (one year older) brother Sigfrid in a student's cap coming down the hill. Soon this brother declares he is going to kiss Sara on the mouth. She reminds him that she is "secretly engaged" to Isak. But after a while he suddenly kisses her "rather skillfully" and is kissed back "with a certain fierceness." Now she cries desperately, pointing to all the spilled strawberries and, especially (and rather symbolically), to a red spot on her dress. Thus Isak obviously made himself relive events typical for his crisis of intimacy (versus isolation)—a crisis decisive in late adolescence and in young adulthood. On the outcome of that crisis, we have claimed, depends much of the ripening capacity for love. (And indeed, we have heard Isak already testify to the unhappiness of his marriage.)

The Summerhouse

But now his daydreaming for that is what we call such mixtures of open-eyed dreams and memories (here made very dramatic and beautiful by what the cinema can do with it all)—makes Isak reach even further back into his childhood. No words can match what Bergman can do, when he suddenly lets the at first "sleepy" facade of a house come alive, with a Swedish-Norwegian flag above it all, and a gong suddenly bringing to life a large number of people, all ready for breakfast. Isak, invisible in his own dream, remains a distant stranger in this "new old world." He hears somebody say that he is out fishing with his father, and he feels a "completely inexplicable happiness in this." But his brothers and sisters are all there, along with an aunt who apparently is the loud and commanding head of the household and its law and order; and there is also old (and seemingly somewhat childish) Uncle Aron, whose birthday it is. A couple of redheaded twin sisters ("as identical as two wild strawberries") in loud unison announce the secrets of the day, among them the fact that Sigfrid had kissed Sara, whereupon Sara runs sobbing out into the hall, where she tells a sister who wants to help her that, yes, Isak was "so enormously refined" and "extremely intellectual," but that he would kiss her only in the dark.

Inside the dining room, though, the vitally gay and yet very orderly breakfast culminates in a festive acknowledgment of Uncle Aron's birthday. The twins have composed a song and now sing it for the totally deaf man. At the end, the aunt suggests a quadruple cheer. All hurrah. And then they seem to see Isak's father appear in the window. That, apparently, is too much for the dreamer himself; abruptly, Isak stands alone, now back where he was: at the wild-strawberry patch with a "feeling of emptiness and sadness"—of despair, maybe?

The Modern "Children"

Suddenly, as if she had jumped from a tree, a most real and modern young lady in shorts and a boy's checked shirt stands there: She is "very tanned," and her blond hair is "tangled and bleached by the sun and the sea." She sucks on an unlit pipe and wears "wooden sandals on her feet and dark glasses on her nose." And she asks him whether the yellow house is *his* shack and the car by the gate *his* jalopy. Her name is (yes) Sara, and she is on her way to Italy. Dr. Borg, enjoying their conversation, declares without hesitation that he would be "honored" if she came along to Lund in his car. Then Marianne reappears and joins his amused welcome: and this collaborative care for a youngster made for the "first contact" between them. As they go back to the car, however, they find two young men, obviously Sara's co-wanderers, waiting, and Isak tells them, "Just jump in." As it turns out, they are young men in training: Victor for a medical degree and Anders for the ministry. In driving on and in looking at them, and especially her, in his rearview mirror, Dr. Borg tells this new Sara of the old Sara, his first love, who is now seventy-five; the modern Sara says she cannot think of "anything worse than getting old"—and then abjectly apologizes. Then, by way of introduction, she humorously declares herself a virgin trying to decide which young man to marry. Here one must remember the role that the sun of Italy then played in the search for identity of young northerners. The conversation makes it clear that the studies assigned to the two young men underscored two conflicting ideologies, a scientific and a religious one, and her choice of one of them will obviously to a large extent determine her identity, as a doctor's or a minister's future wife, and thus her fidelity — the personal strength emanating from a solution of one's identity struggle. For the trip, however, the young men have agreed not to argue about science or about God. And so, this new generation of passengers adds to the stages of life that old Dr. Borg must apparently still come to terms with—his choice of a professional identity as a doctor—before he can truly face the existential identity of old age. All this will be played out significantly and even enjoyably later during the drive.

The Accident

Steadily ahead, then, is the country road. At a moment still full of laughter over Sara's sincere repentance because of her remark on aging, Isak, in trying to negotiate a blind curve, suddenly sees a little black car coming right at them. As both cars jam on their brakes, "ours" goes safely off the road into a pasture, while the other one, overturning, falls into a ditch. A middle-aged couple climb out of it, miraculously unhurt, but continuing a quarrel that apparently caused the mishap in the first place. In meeting Dr. Borg, they take full responsibility for the accident: the woman, who was driving, confesses that she was about to slap her husband when it happened. But now they continue to make bitter fun of each other, especially in regard to their ideological position in life: in no time, she refers to him as a "Catholic," and he calls her a "genius at hysterics" and a believer in psychotherapy: both ideological failures, maybe—and thus an incompatibility?

The young men and the husband succeed in turning the little car right side up, but then one front wheel rolls off: "A true picture of our marriage," remarks the wife. Well, Isak asks them to come along (on the folding chairs), to the next gas station. Once in the car, however, the wife starts to sob, and her husband makes such indiscreet fun of her that Marianne asks him to leave her alone. But he continues his disdainful attacks until his wife suddenly slaps his face. At that moment, Marianne slowly but definitely stops the car and, pointing to a nearby house where there might be a telephone, tells them to get out—for the children's sake. In our terms: her sense of care does not permit her to let such careless and uncaring behavior continue in the presence of the young. Here she speaks up for everybody's parenthood. Alman, from the roadside, apologizes quite downheartedly. The drive continues.

Midday, Midlife

As midday is reached, so, apparently, is Isak's midlife: and here we really learn of "*Dr.* Borg." Everybody now needs fresh supplies, beginning with the vehicle that carries them across the map—and the stages of life. So they stop at a gas station, which proves to be well selected. The strong blond owner, Åkerman, immediately recognizes Dr. Borg and assumes that the occupants of the car are his children and grandchildren; but he also confesses to have been a patient, from his birth on, of the "world's best doctor"—as were all his brothers and as was his wife, Eva, who is described as beaming "like a big strawberry in her red dress." This seems to be a significant variation of the movie's title, for Eva is indeed pregnant, and Åkerman then and there suggests that they call the baby Isak (they have only sons). Is our Isak going to be a godfather before he becomes a grandfather? But here we are reminded that what we call generativity can, in different lives, be fulfilled by different ratios of procreative, productive, and creative services to mankind. And it makes Isak very thoughtful to be in that noon hour in that part of Sweden, apparently a landscape with a "wide view" and "rich foliage." And so he whispers to himself (possibly not without being heard by Åkerman) that perhaps he "should have remained here," in such a small community, where he apparently practiced medicine for fifteen years and is now

remembered by everyone as a doctor who truly "cared"—
that is, before he became more academic: a not atypical old
man's mourning for an abandoned part of his identity.

The Pensive Meal

For lunch, the occupants of the car face each other around
a large table on the open terrace of a nearby inn with a
magnificent view. Their waiter, too, was once Dr. Borg's
patient. The doctor, with the help of some wine, tells anecdotes "of human interest," and they are "a great success."
Eventually, Anders rises to recite a poem on the Creation
and its Creator, whereupon Viktor reminds him of their
forbidden subjects—and there they go again: rationalism versus religion. But Sara is touched by Anders's recital and says
that she always agrees with the one of the two "sweet boys"
who has spoken last. Isak keeps still, but in the next moment,
just after Marianne lights his cigar, he begins to recite something, too. It begins, "Where is the friend I seek everywhere?
Dawn is the time of loneliness and care," and it ends with
the help of both Anders and Marianne: "In every sign and
breath of air, His love is there." To which Sara remarks,
"You're religious, aren't you, Professor?"

We will return to this scene. But if we related its pensive-
ness to the whole course of life, we would have to say that
the religiosity maturing in old age contains a need for a belief
in an ultimate other whose logos reveals itself in human life.
Viktor, the rationalist, seems to have an inkling of this as
much as does the monotheist Anders, for it is at the end of
adolescence and the beginning of young adulthood that such
figures of a significant other can be represented by charismatic leaders or creative voices as well as by gods. Such
shared others are a necessary counterpart to the sense of "I"
and of "we" that matures in adolescence.

But here we must repeat that, developmentally speaking, the lifelong sense of "I" and of "We" first emerges at the very beginning of life out of the bonding experience of the mother (or the significant maternal person), whom we therefore call the primal other. And so, the scene by Lake Vättern makes all the more "sense" when Isak, after a long silence, abruptly announces that he now will visit his mother, who lives nearby. Marianne declares she would like to come along.

The Mother Revisited

As we turn from the lakeside scene and its ultimate perspectives to a revisitation of Isak's mother, now nearly a hundred years old, we must notice, besides—or, rather, within—the great drama, those smallest gestures of which Bergman is such a master. We noticed that, just before Isak's recital, Marianne lit his cigar for him. Now, on the way to the mother's house, Marianne takes his arm and he pats her hand: truly, for such proud individuals, gestures expressing some mutual trust. But—and how often Bergman makes us introduce a new scene with *but*—when it comes into view, the mother's house proves to be surrounded by a stone wall "as tall as a man"; inside, everything seems somewhat unreal, like a set in an old theater. The mother is dressed all in black. She seems well aware of his "great day," and greets her son "with both her hands stretched forth"—and he kisses them. *But* when she sees Marianne, she wonders whether that is his wife and, if so, whether she should "leave the room immediately. . . . She has hurt us too much." Corrected, she wants to know why Marianne is not at home ("with her child").

Now she points to a large box, which Marianne brings to her: it proves to be filled with old toys, and she seems to know to which of her children and grandchildren each toy once belonged. But for a frightening moment does she not seem to find the children themselves in the box rather than their toys and things? Then she enumerates her offspring: ten children, only Isak alive. Twenty grandchildren, and only Evald visits her—once a year. Of her (God knows how many) great-grandchildren, she has never met fifteen. She must remember fifty-three birthdays and anniversaries every year. Her great fault, she now concludes, is that she has not died, for everybody is waiting for her money—certainly a frequent, if not always confessed, trend of mind among the oldest. At any rate, as some thunder rumbles, she concludes that it does not "pay much to talk." In fact, she asks, "Isn't it cold in here?" and adds, "I've always felt chilly as long as I can remember. What does that mean? You're a doctor? Mostly in the stomach. Here." Soberly, Dr. Borg blames her chill on her low blood pressure.

As they get ready to leave, the mother requests their advice concerning just one last item in the box: her father's gold watch. And, yes, the dial is handless! Isak thinks of his deadly dream of the night before, but then the visit ends with an episode indicative of some trust and caring: the mother trusts that the watch can be repaired, for she wants to give it to her grandchild Sigbritt's boy, who will be fifty soon. And Isak, having kissed his mother good-bye, notes that her face is very cold but "unbelievably soft" and "full of sharp little lines." She has lived a long life. As they walk away from the place, Marianne again takes Isak's arm and he "is filled with gratitude toward this quiet, independent girl."

Three Dreams

When they return to their car, Isak and Marianne find an utterly disgusted Sara close to tears: the boys, down the hill, are still "slugging it out" about their ideological ultimates: Couldn't they "skip God and pay some attention" to her? But soon they are all back in the car, with Marianne at the wheel. The sleepy Isak blesses his luck in having her beside him as a reliable chauffeur. Now he can take a nap—but not without a series of dreams—"extremely real and very humiliating" to him.

In recording these dreams in his diary, Dr. Borg denies "the slightest intention of commenting on their possible meaning," and states his attitude toward such matters: "I have never been particularly enthusiastic about the psychoanalytical theory of dreams as the fulfillment of desires in a negative or positive direction. Yet I cannot deny that in these dreams there was something like a warning, which bore into my consciousness and embedded itself there with relentless determination." Involvement, then! And he adds, "I have found that during the last few years I glide rather easily into a twilight world of memories and dreams which are highly personal. I've often wondered if this is a sign of increasing senility. Sometimes I've also asked myself if it is a harbinger of approaching death."

These reflections of Dr. Borg happen to correspond to some of Bergman's own opinions as expressed in the introduction of the book of screenplays from which we are quoting here. There Bergman states, "Philosophically, there is a book which was a tremendous experience for me: Eiono Kailn's *Psychology of the Personality*. His thesis that man lives strictly according to his needs —negative and positive — was shattering to me, but terribly true. And I built on this ground." All this may seem to call for some methodological discussion on our part; but nobody is being "psychoanalyzed" in our account. We are using a great work in order to find in its dramatic dynamics a confirmation and a guide in our attempt to formulate some of the developmental logos of the stages of life as we have come to chart them in an expansion of psychoanalytic thought. In their own dramatic logic, the doctor's dreams seem to make deeply "life-historical" sense (as he realizes without the help of any psychoanalyst), for as it takes him back to the strawberry patch near the old family house, and (in a moment) to his classroom in medical school, we will see that deep down he is aware of the distant rigidity of which Marianne accused him: Does he begin to realize that in his old age he must yet relax the kind of forced integrity that has characterized his very first self-description? But dreams are visual experiences par excellence, and here they are dramatic scenes as well. So we can only attempt to state in brief summaries what Isak seems to be trying to tell himself by making his own dream figures confront him.

1. Back at the wild-strawberry patch, Sara is sitting near Isak, and a little basket full of wild strawberries is between them. She looks at him for a long time and then speaks to him in a grieved and penetrating tone that he can hardly hear. Has he ever looked at himself in a mirror? She pulls one out from under the basket and makes him face himself. How old he is; and he must die soon, whereas she has a lifetime before her. Now he seems offended, she continues, for he cannot bear the truth. She has been too considerate with him. He only *thinks* he understands. "Look at yourself in the mirror," she says, then tells him that she is about to marry Sigfrid. He should try to smile. "It hurts." She concludes, "You, a professor emeritus, ought to know why it hurts. But you don't. Because in spite of all your knowledge you don't really know anything." Sara throws away the mirror, and it shatters. Through all this, he sits there knowing that he is old, ugly, ridiculous. He, the Jubilee Doctor, can only stam-

mer when he tries to answer her. She cannot hear his words; but "they don't really matter."

Then, a baby cries somewhere. Sara arises. She had "promised to look after Sigbritt's little boy," and, ignoring Isak's plea not to leave him, she runs up to the arbor and cradles the child: "My poor little one, you shall sleep quietly now. Don't be afraid of the wind. Don't be afraid of the birds, the jackdaws and the sea gulls. Don't be afraid of the waves from the sea. I'm with you. I'm holding you tight. Don't be afraid, little one. Soon it will be another day. No one can hurt you; I am with you; I'm holding you." All this time, she cries. And Isak wants to scream until his lungs are bloody.

At the end of Isak's visit to his mother, we remember, Sigbritt's now grown-up boy was going to get from Isak's mother her father's watch—repaired. Here, Sara takes care of Sigbritt's boy. Does the Sara of this dream remind him of the mother he himself experienced when he was an infant— and she was young? But, of course, he had lost *her,* as any infant loses the primal other when he grows up and watches her motherliness directed toward the subsequent children.

There follows a dream scene at the door of the house behind the patch: Sigfrid is calling Sara, and she, with the baby, runs to him. The "blackened" day begins to clear, and there is piano music. Isak presses his face against the window, as he sees a mature and formally clad Sara share a festive dinner *à deux.* Isak taps on the window but is not heard. Somehow he cuts a hand: the cut looks like a stigmatization. Needless to say, the dream dramatizes again the sense of isolation that is the dystonic counterpart to the intimacy that Isak has missed so much as a man.

2. With the power of a blinding moonlight, the dream now changes totally. The same door opens on another scene, and there stands a frigid Mr. Alman. We saw him last, standing

by that roadside ("like a schoolboy who had been scolded") apologizing for his and his wife's atrocious behavior. Now he is, apparently, himself a kind of judge, an examiner who, politely and stiffly, invites Isak to his old polyclinical lecture-and-examination amphitheater. There is a totally still audience of youngsters, including Anders and Viktor with *their* Sara. Having studied Isak's examination book, and (he too) having silently looked at him for a long time, Alman gestures him to a microscope and asks him to identify a bacteriological specimen. All Dr. Borg can see in the microscope is his own "absurdly enlarged" eye: "I can't see anything." Then Alman points to the blackboard and asks him to read something printed on it in large but "foreign" letters. Dr. Borg cannot read it. Alman reads it for him—"A doctor's first duty is to ask forgiveness"—and now concludes, "You are guilty of guilt." (Does this mean sin?)

Throughout all this, Dr. Borg tries to find excuses: the microscope is no good; he is a doctor, not a linguist; and now he claims that he is an old man with a bad heart. But the examiner declares that there is nothing about Isak's heart in his books and continues, lighting a lamp over the face of a woman (Mrs. Alman) and asking him to diagnose her. Dr. Borg declares the patient to be dead—and she laughs loudly about it as a great joke. Alman's overall conclusion in regard to the examination is "That you're incompetent." The Jubilee Doctor!

But then he adds that Isak also was accused of "indifference, selfishness, lack of consideration"—and all this by his wife! Dr. Borg's final excuse: she is long dead. But Alman asks him to come along and leads him into a forest.

3. In the light of a moon resembling an "inflamed eye," Alman and he enter a world of dead trees, oozing mud, a porous ground, and snakes. The scene that follows (how much of it is memory, how much dream?) seems to reveal,

with all dramatic means, what a foreigner Isak is and how hysterical his wife was in matters of passion: in that forest "where snakes seemed to well forth from the swampy, porous ground," we hear a woman's giggling gradually turning into uncontrollable laughter as she flails the air in trying to escape the advances of a virile but somehow disgusting man —a man who "tries to pull the pins out of her hair" and speaks to her "as if to an animal" while she is "crying, rocking, and swaying." Suddenly, she is completely still, as she "receives" him "between her knees." Then they sit there, he with his cigar and she thinking what would (or will) happen if she told Isak about this. He will say, she predicts, "You shouldn't ask forgiveness from me. I have nothing to forgive." And again, "But would he ever *ask* for forgiveness?" She may accuse him of a "sickening" nobility, and he will offer her a sedative, claiming that he understands.

Then Isak dreams that Alman calls his dreams "a surgical masterpiece," for "everything has been dissected"—a "perfect achievement of its kind." Dr. Borg asks what the penalty is. He is told, "Loneliness, of course." "Is there no grace?" he asks. But *that* his examiner does not claim to know. And then he disappears.

4. There is one more brief scene where Sara once more "materializes." "If only you had stayed with me" is all he can say. He tries to follow her, but she moves "so much more easily and faster" than he. And then she, too, is gone. So is the moon. And Isak wants to cry with "wild, childish sorrow."

The Son's Despair

On awakening, Isak finds himself in the car alone with Marianne, in another beautiful Swedish countryside. The children "are out picking flowers" for him, the jubileer.

"Good Lord!" he says. But he uses their moment alone to tell Marianne about his dreaming: "It's as if I'm trying to say something to myself which I don't want to hear when I'm awake." To her question "And what would that be?" he answers, "That I am dead, although I live." To this she reacts violently: "Do you know that you and Evald are very much alike?"

Isak: "You told me that."

Marianne: "Do you know that Evald has said the very same thing?"

Isak: "About me? Yes, I can believe that."

Marianne: "No, about himself."

Isak: "But he's only thirty-eight years old."

Marianne: "May I tell you everything, or would it bore you?"

At last!

Just before she came to visit him, Marianne had wanted to tell Evald something and, as we now witness, had driven him to the beach, the sea "merging with clouds in infinite grayness." "So now you have me trapped," Evald admits and wonders whether her secret is another man. No, she says, "I'm pregnant," and adds, "I shall have this child." They both feel cold. After sitting "quietly for a long time" and "whistling soundlessly," Evald marches through the rain down to the beach and stands under a tree for another while. Finally, she goes to him, and he says (icily, calmly, it seems) that she must choose between him and the child: he cannot accept what may force him "to exist another day longer than he wants." He thinks he was an unwelcome child, and is Isak sure he is his son? She tries to tell him that his attitude is wrong. And here it comes again:

"There is nothing," Evald says, "which can be called right or wrong. One functions according to one's needs; you can read that in an elementary-school textbook."

Marianne: "And what do we need?"

Evald: "You have a damned need to live, to exist and create life."

Marianne: "And how about you?"

Evald: "My need is to be dead. Absolutely, totally dead."

This is Marianne's story. All Isak can do is ask her whether she wants to smoke. And smoking helps her confess that she finds his mother's ice-cold state of mind "more frightening than death itself"; and now Isak declares himself dead while living, and Evald is just about to. But she says, "I want my child; nobody can take it from me. Not even the person I love more than anyone else." (She will not stand for generational death, then.) Isak records that Marianne's gaze at this point was "black, accusing, desperate": "I suddenly felt shaken in a way which I had never experienced before." But what he says is simply "Can I help you?"—which is what she hoped to hear in the first place, when she came to visit him. So here, at last, a latent theme decisive for this whole drama has come into the open. You may remember that in that very first dream, we seemed to hear a baby's cries right in the swaying and rocking noise made by the hearse; this meant to us (and I hope, to Bergman) that the doctor in Isak could not help being at least intuitively aware of Marianne's pregnancy, even if he was too "dead" then, to face it. But much has happened since then to revive the Borgs.

On to Lund

And now it is time to drive to Lund. Marianne blows the horn and starts the motor. The children appear with a large bouquet of wildflowers, and Sara solemnly hands them to Isak through the car window, declaring how impressed they are that he is so old and has been a doctor for so long: "one who knows all about life and who has learned all the prescriptions by heart," whereupon she curtsies and kisses him on the cheek. Then they all board for the last stretch of the trip.

As they arrive at Evald's house, everybody is there waiting, but Isak first notices "a small, round woman," Agda: so she had made it by plane. And though she still is somewhat sour ("the fun is gone"), she proves to have played her preparatory role most efficiently. Evald is all dressed up for the ceremony and the dinner: *he* is pleased to see Marianne, who, when asked whether she wants a room in the hotel, asks, "Why?" and proves ready to share Evald's bedroom "for one more night." And yes, she will go to the dinner, too. We thus face, on that last day of our visit there, a whole series of the simplest and most sensible personal and generational encounters, of the kind that also make this dynamic movie a stage for an ordinary display and interplay of all human emotions. At the end, they are made only more convincing by this very special, ceremonial day.

Now they all drive to Lund's beautiful ancient cathedral (more recently, Hammarskjöld was buried there). Let Dr. Borg describe the overall setting: "Trumpet fanfares, bells ringing, field-cannon salutes, masses of people, the giant procession from the university to the cathedral, the white-dressed garland girls, royalty, old age, wisdom, beautiful music, stately Latin sentences which echoed off the huge vaults. The students and their girls, women in bright, magnificent dresses, this strange rite with its heavy symbolism." Isak, in a most dignified way, goes through the ceremonial motions, delightedly seeing "the children" in the applauding crowd and Agda and Marianne in the invited audience. He really continues thinking of the "day just lived (and dreamt) through" and concludes that there is a "remarkable reality in this chain of unexpected untangled events," while all the noisy festivities now seem "as meaningless as a passing dream!" But soon he, too, stands at the altar—top spot of it all—to be crowned with that famous black hat.

Day's End

For the banquet, however, he is too tired, so he takes a taxi home. There Agda has everything prepared for the good night that he needs; and he feels great warmth for her. So, as she helps him undress, the new honorary doctor does ask for forgiveness: "I'm sorry for this morning." She responds, "Are you sick, Professor?" After a while, he, even more daringly suggests that maybe it is time that they address each other with *"du"*—which would correspond in the English-speaking world to the mutual use of first names. But she wonders what people would say and, anyway, begs to be "excused from all intimacies." Retiring, she leaves her door ajar, in case he wants something.

Lying down to sleep, Isak hears musical noises and, indeed, getting up once more, sees the "children" down in the garden, singing and guitarring. Then Sara loudly voices the truly final word: "Goodbye, Father Isak. Do you know that it is really you I love, today, tomorrow and forever?" Isak replies, "I'll remember that."

Then Evald and Marianne come home for a moment, because she has broken a heel. Isak calls Evald in and asks what is going to happen between them.

Evald: "I have asked her to remain with me."

Isak: "And how will it . . . I mean . . ."

Evald: "I can't be without her."

Isak: "You mean you can't live alone?"

Evald: "I can't be without *her.* That's what I mean."

Isak: "I understand."

Evald: "It will be as she wants."

But a remark regarding his loan (remember?) is misunderstood by Evald, who assures Isak that he will get his money back. Then Marianne comes to sit on his bed for a moment, and Isak's senses seem to have been activated by it all, for he notes that she "smelled good and rustled in a sweet, womanly way." To her, he says only, "I like you," and she declares, "I like you, too, Father Isak." And yet what essential matters have been settled between them—and their generations!

Finally, alone, Isak "hears" his heart and his old watch, and the tower clock, as it strikes eleven: one hour before midnight. But there occurs one more—what? The technical term would be *daydream,* for it is a dream that one might well have while awake. Here, however, the dreamer happens to be awake near midnight, and Isak, when recording it, feels that he must explain. Whenever he is restless or sad, he tries *now,* he tells us, to "recall memories of his childhood to calm down." That night, he wanders back again to the summer-house and the strawberry patch and to everything that he "dreamed or remembered or experienced" that day. It sounds like a visual lullaby that he now imagines; a "warm, sunny day" with "a mild breeze coming through the birches." Down at the dock, his sisters and brothers are romping with Uncle Aron and applauding when the red sail goes up. Now Sara passes by and, seeing him, comes running and says, "Isak, darling, there are no wild strawberries left. Aunt wants you to search for your father. We will sail around the peninsula and pick you up on the other side."

Isak: "I have already searched for him, but I can't find either Father or Mother."

Sara: "Your mother was supposed to go with him."

Isak: "Yes, but I can't find them."

Sara: "I will help you."

And Sara now takes him by the hand and leads him to "a narrow sound with deep, dark water."

What Isak sees there is his father fishing and his mother reading a book, as distant from each other as these activities demanded. When Sara sees that he has noticed his parents she drops his hand and suddenly is gone, obviously leaving him to his own experience of ultimate or, rather, primary recognition.

What we really mean to suggest here is that one's sense of "I," which is the center of our awareness, is first experienced in infancy when the mother is recognized as a recognizable "you": thus, she becomes, as we have said, the primal other in our life. There is a limited series of other "others" throughout life, beginning with the father, who thus can contribute an ideal model for such father figures as charismatic leaders and, of course, God. At any rate, Isak, after having looked for a long time at the pair, tries to shout but "not a sound" comes from his mouth. All this is, incidentally, described in terms of the historical time: his father is dressed like a gentleman fisherman and the mother wears a big hat. At last the father sees him and waves, laughing; and the mother looks up from her book, also laughs—and nods.

It all ends thus: "I dreamed that I stood by the water and shouted toward the bay, but the warm summer breeze carried away my cries and they did not reach their destination. yet I wasn't sorry about that; I felt, on the contrary, rather lighthearted."

One cannot help hoping that Isak's lightheartedness is in the service of the peaceful sleep we think he has deserved after that day. But we also hope that the total experience of the day we witnessed will eventually see him somewhat more "reinvolved" in human life than he appears to be in his initial self-description. For what could have caused in him the day-long experience of such a self-confrontation, if not a wish for some involvement? We believe that this was caused by a combination of the celebration and of Marianne's pregnancy, in addition to some kind of age-specific spiritual readiness; none of this seems to be sufficiently expressed in the kind of withdrawn wisdom and compulsive integrity that character-ize the original introduction to his diary. At any rate, Ma-rianne's now-generative passion and her true caring demanded of Isak's self-confrontation more than an "ad-justment" to his old condition, and more than an accep-tance of *reality:* we call *actuality* what reinvolved him and those closest to him that day, as became so clear in the simplest and yet also most "related" interactions of the final scenes.

Or, maybe, too, there is a problem of historical relativity in all this: the historical period in which Dr. Borg reached old age makes it still quite plausible that he, as such a rare survivor in his family and in his community, should be some-thing of a classical elder with a withdrawn integrity and with something of a pseudo-integrity like the one he describes, but today one wonders what more *vital involvement* in private and in communal affairs could be expected of such a man. (Lund Physicians for Social Responsibility?) Maybe, also, we can trust Marianne to continue insisting that even at his age he develop somewhat of a grandparental generativity both in personal affairs and in the community. It may, in fact, just be that fate was waiting for a daughter figure to take on the generational role in the Borg family and to teach both of these astonished doctors something about father-hood.

2. Isak's Stages

In the preceding section, we reviewed Bergman's film scene by scene, indicating which stage of Dr. Borg's life cycle is being relived by him in the service of reremembering his life story in terms of his old age. It may now be clarifying for us to indicate explicitly, at the risk of being somewhat repetitious, how his "restored" life history permits us to reconstruct the various stages of life as first lived by the growing and maturing Isak. Let us see, in fact, how Dr. Borg expresses in his own words the tensions between the syntonic and dystonic aspects of each stage as well as the strength then to be fostered. We will turn to the original script for clarifying details and for the English version of the Swedish dialogue.

First we must remind ourselves that Dr. Borg is still alive at the end of the film and as a legendary figure remains for us immortal. He is only falling asleep peacefully at the end of the last scene. The tension between the syntonic and dystonic pulls will, then, continue for him, and, indeed, he can continue to develop new strengths if favorable experiences offer themselves and if he is ready and able to accept change —and age.

It is also good to remember that the entire story of *Wild Strawberries* is based on Dr. Borg's own journal, which, he tells us, he began to write on the day after his trip to Lund. One of the remarkable aspects of this account, however, is the devotion to the experiential detail, the sensual, exact description of sound, sight, touch, and even taste and smell. Such perceptive acuity is rare in didactic accounts, being found outstandingly as an attribute of the work of the artists of the world. There it must be an integral element in the expression of all the art forms. The artistry of Bergman's Dr.

Borg is apparent in the choice of his words. He was, after all, a professor, an esteemed teacher. His field was bacteriology, which demands exactness and attention to detail. As an adolescent and very young man, he also found pleasure in the reading of poetry, an enthusiasm he wanted to share with his young cousin Sara.

He tells us that for the first twenty years of his life he spent the summers at the house on the shore with his siblings and cousins. It was apparently a stimulating, unusually lively environment. The early years of our old doctor, about whose childhood we otherwise know very little, were thus, we can assume, rich with sensory experience. These enlivening exposures to natural stimuli are enduring and remain acute components of memory long after fact and number have for many become vague and perhaps unimportant. The poems of elderly persons have repeatedly demonstrated this persistence of sensory memory. It may be a vital component of all daydreaming in old age. At any rate, Dr. Borg's dreams and half-waking fantasies are exceptionally vivid in every sensory detail. We can appreciate this lively involvement in his environs as we follow him from one stage to another.

Infancy

Since we posit hope as the first basic strength to be nurtured in infancy—a strength that in its turn supports all the earliest as well as the future development of the individual —let us now consider the matrix into which this particular child, Isak Borg, was born. We would assume that the matrix is naturally made up of the environs and the caretakers. How much does the film story reveal to us of the space in which Isak spent his first years? The summerhouse and its spacious and desirable location suggest that the family winter home must have been more than adequately upper bourgeois. One would imagine a nursery used in turn by the ten children as they arrived. Isak, one assumes, was physically well taken care of. Babies are not born equal in physical endowment, but Isak was probably a husky infant who grew into an aging man in apparent good health. In any case, he outlived all his siblings.

His mother, who one assumes was his primary caretaker, gives every evidence of being a physically exceptional woman, having produced ten children and remained very much in charge of her life. The gas station attendant speaks of her, at ninety-six years of age, as "a miracle of health and vitality." But she is cool and distant and states explicitly, "I've *always* felt chilly." However, Dr. Borg tells Marianne a surprisingly observed detail about her that reinforces our earlier suggestion. He says of his mother, "Her senses are as sharp as those of an animal in the woods." This kind of sensory acuity would have been a component of the mutuality of shared experiences between infant and mother and may have provided early stimulation for this child. Babies were usually delivered at home in those days and breast-fed, if not by the mother then by a wet nurse. It is thus reasonable to assume that for a year or so his senses—touch, smell, and taste, as well as sight and hearing—were actively involved in his milieu.

It is not clear in the story how many older and/or younger siblings Isak had. However, in the birthday scene some of the children seem very young; yet although he is the only survivor he is not the oldest, since his mother speaks disparagingly of his older brother. Did his young mother have time to devote to this perhaps middle son, time to be playful with him, or was he well washed and bedded and left a good deal to himself?

We are justified in assuming that orderliness played an important role in this family. Even in the summer vacation house, schedule was the rule. Clocks are an important image in his dreams, and even when he is an old man his mother shows him his father's faceless watch, a gift to be given to her oldest grandson, aged fifty, on his expected visit to her. Cleanliness, we may also suppose, is highly valued in this milieu. The aunt in the birthday party scene makes a great point of clean hands and fingernails at the table, and young Sara's distress over her stained dress is further evidence of this valuing.

In fact, one senses in general some shared communal and firmly held values that stress schedules, deportment, and decency. This is probably not a matrix that could bend easily to respond to even the loud protest of an infant needing, for whatever reason, special evidence of mutuality and sensory nourishment. One senses that in this early period Isak may have needed somewhat more warm, flexible mothering and sensitive caring than he got.

At the very opening of the film, Dr. Borg describes himself by saying quite clearly, "All I ask of life is to be left alone" —a sweeping statement of withdrawal. There will be some evidence of this tendency throughout the story, as we proceed through his life stages, but there are also a number of themes suggesting trustfulness in his life.

We believe one can clearly see in his memory of the young Sara and of the older Sara and in his immediate response to the modern Sara a reevoking of the longing for the mutuality of his early relationship with his own young mother. This youthful feminine character reappears often and dominates the story—but always walks away.

Furthermore, as an expression of some deep-lying sense of trust and hope, there is Dr. Borg's introduction of the song

at the luncheon party with the youngsters and Marianne—
a poem that is a hymn of faith and is well known to her and
Anders, the young theologian.

He recites:

Where is the friend I seek everywhere?
Dawn is the time of loneliness and care.

Anders continues:

When twilight comes I am still yearning
Though my heart is burning, burning.
I see his trace of glory and power
In an ear of grain and the fragrance of a flower

And Marianne ends:

In every sign and breath of air
His love is there.

The revelatory experiences of the day's trip, it seems, have
moved this old man deeply, for later, at the ceremony in
Lund, he ruminates about the day, planning to recollect and
write down everything that happened. He says, "I was beginning to see a remarkable causality in this chain of unexpected, entangled events." Is such causality not an article of
scientific faith? And later, in the final scene, he stands by the
water and shouts toward his parents, who are far away and
involved in their own affairs (as usual?). They fish and read
on an opposite bank and do not respond except with a slight,
waved greeting. Yet their very presence, even at such a distance, must have been reassuring for their last surviving son.
He says, "Yet I wasn't sorry about that. I felt on the contrary
rather lighthearted." In fact, he goes to sleep smiling peacefully.

The whole picture, then, actually ends on a note of hope.

Indeed, in the final scenes at least some essential reconciliation with his son is promised. Even Marianne's simple "I like you too, Father Isak," is a gift from this determined young woman whose faith in generativity he has learned to prize and respect. And, of course, there is the vitalizing promise of a grandchild.

Early Childhood

With the second stage, which introduces the development of musculature and experiments with independence, the environs as well as the relationships of the toddler expand. We really see Isak Borg only as an old man. He is present as observer in all the scenes of which he must have been a part in his youth. But he moves freely, if with appropriate caution, for he knows well that in old age it is contraindicated to fall—doctors know that old bones are brittle and break all too easily.

No longer confined to restricted safe spaces, to crib or playpen, the toddler may explore larger environs and becomes a more involved member of the family—joining siblings, aunts, uncles, and cousins. And the Borg family was obviously an extended one, whose members shared at least their summers. This offers many challenges for a youngster, such as older figures to admire and emulate, but also competitors and persons to be jealous of.

The demands on a toddler are also more severe. This is the period for bowel training and the struggle with caretakers as to how and when and where these eliminating functions may take place. And there are penalties for defying the social norms that the adults impose. Shaming is the device used most freely by families to enforce social rules, and name-calling is resorted to with implications of lack of control, uncleanness, gluttony, selfishness, carelessness. This kind of shaming can be weathered if there is also adequate supportive encouragement and some good humor. More deeply injurious are the doubts and aspersions that the youngster encounters from older siblings and adults concerning the adequacy of actual physical or mental capacities.

Throughout this period, keen sensory awareness can support in the child a true and appropriate sense of available abilities so that a strong willfulness may be maintained along with a social compliance, which also offers its rewards.

It would appear that Isak throughout his childhood struggled perhaps stubbornly or even rebelliously to exert his right to be himself. He is in his old age a very independent and strong-willed character with well-defined inflexibility and some presumption.

The young Sara may be expressing the extended family's characterization of young Isak when she bewails his "fine ness," his "intellectuality," and his wanting only to "read poetry" with her. Perhaps it is his "difference," a solitariness, that sets him apart and appeals to her idealism.

As an old man, however, Dr. Borg speaks out his plans and wishes very decisively. Following his nightmare dream at the beginning of the film, Dr. Borg awakens at 3:00 A.M. He says, "I knew immediately what I should do." He then wakens Agda and tells her, "I'm taking the car . . . I'll drive down to Lund with my own two hands." He is seventy-six years old, and the drive to Lund takes fourteen hours. He plans to go alone. Agda, equally strong-willed, and he then spar, which he cuts off with, "We are not married, Miss Agda. . . . I'm a grown man and I don't have to put up with your bossiness." No reticence here. He is master of his house and of himself.

Miss Agda and he have together successfully provided him

with excellent physical care—he is vital, strong, and willful. But an underlying shame, doubt, and confusion are clearly manifested in the dream scene with the inquisitor when he is examined. He defends himself by trying to evade responsibility for this medical matter since his professional acumen is at stake. "There is something wrong with the microscope." "I'm a doctor, not a linguist." Finally, when his bravado fails, he pleads almost childishly, "I'm an old man and must be treated with consideration."

The theme of early-childhood shame as experienced in old age is most painfully expressed when the older Sara forces him in a dream scene to look in the mirror she offers him and shows him his face, which looks "old and ugly." She follows this by saying, "In spite of all your knowledge you don't really know anything," another telling blow to his intellectual pride. This dream theme is, no doubt, suggested by the way Marianne unhesitatingly confronts him.

He boasts readily of his relationship with his son. They are very much alike, he claims, and understand one another in an intelligent, practical way. However, his face looks stricken when she replies to this cool information with the indictment "That may be true, but he also hates you." She seems to respect this strong, controlled old man but also to recognize the destructive quality of the ruthless willfulness with which the son has been obliged to contend.

Play Age

The third stage is the age of play, and the child's matrix of being includes not only the extended family and close friends, peers, and playmates but also the environs of the play school or kindergarten. Games, fairy tales, and songs stimulate the imagination and open the doors to vicarious experience. Inventiveness and initiative are offered free play, but within limits that protect the space and rights of others. The overstepping of these limits is frowned upon by the milieu and the offender is made to feel guilty. By way of an active imagination, one learns to empathize with the sensibilities of others and be respectful of their purposefulness.

It is imperative at this third stage to establish a working relationship with materials and learn to trust their lawfulness and reliability. Mistrust of the world of matter and things is self-limiting and maladaptive. It is also of great importance to become able to differentiate actuality from fantasy by virtue of the reliability of trustworthy sensory experience. Should the fantasy world appear safer than reality, it can become a refuge and result in purposelessness.

How can we visualize Isak at this age relating to the challenges of imaginative play and initiative and coping with restraining social strictures?

We have been aware that throughout the dream fantasy sequences old Dr. Borg is the observer of the youthful scenes. He is apart from the actors and watching a little anxiously but keenly. Only once does he indicate he wants to make himself heard, and at that point he wounds himself on a nail. Perhaps this was the nonparticipator stance he slowly began to assume throughout his childhood. In his differentness, he may have become the visual recorder. His dreams in old age are remarkably vivid, inventive, and minutely recorded in each sensual detail. This role of the observer is a necessary one for the writer and the artist, as well as for the scientist. One wonders throughout about his father as role model, for this is the stage Freud designates as that of the confrontation with the Oedipus complex. Isak's father is seen only once in the film, fishing on the bank of the water—a solitary activity and a very remote figure.

At the beginning of the eventful day we are following, the decision at 3:00 A.M. to drive to Lund seemed both willful and improvised. The story continues in this vein when Dr. Borg decides to turn off and visit the old summerhouse. "Suddenly I had an impulse," he says. There he also quite willingly falls into the plan of taking along first the modern Sara and then her young companions. He initiates the luncheon party with them and is drawn into their squabbles and antics. He is involved, almost playful, and amused. At the bare suggestion of the gas station attendant, his old patient, he apparently decides also to visit his mother, or was this an essential part of his plan in deciding to drive? For some reason, one would not have expected such flexibility from this disciplined old man. The dreams that awakened him seem to have propelled him into asserting his aliveness and self-assertiveness. When Marianne says, "You are an old egotist, Father. . . . you have never listened to anyone but yourself . . . you are hard as nails. . . . We who have seen you at close range, we know what you really are," he tries to laugh off her judgments. When, however, Marianne reacts to his statement "I'm sorry you dislike me" by saying, "I don't dislike you. I feel sorry for you," he is incredulous and again tries to defend himself by claiming to be only amused and noting "her odd tone of voice and lack of logic." This suggests, one senses, a kind of sweeping defense against the judgments of womankind in general.

Later in the dream—when the inquisitor, Alman, forces him to agree, very reluctantly, that "a doctor's first duty is to ask forgiveness"—he acts only stubbornly compliant and confused. When that is followed by the accusation "You are guilty of guilt," all his defenses seem to crumble.

His stance is that of a very humbled man as he then is forced to view again the scene with his wife and her lover in the forest, and as he hears her accusations against him he ages perceptibly—with guilt and shame.

School Age

The development of the basic strength of competence is fostered in every society in the years of schooling. Industriousness is encouraged for the sake of the survival of the individual and of the community. A sense of inferiority, which is its opposite, is adaptive and syntonic only insofar as it provides appropriate modification of any overestimation of capacities. Overestimation of competence can be as maladaptive as underestimation. What is required is accurately perceived capacities, as judged by keen, trustworthy senses.

The school years provide an extended matrix of school and work groups, of teachers, "bosses," of skills carried on outside school and the beginning of a sense of community membership. At this point, trust in one's own tested physical, mental, and social capacities is essential. The earlier experiences with materials, tools, and processes that have been promoted by playful imagination, supported by willpower, and guided by purposefulness reinforce one's approach to all study. But the dystonic also curbs and modifies: mistrust, shame, and guilt are essential so that the individual may avoid egocentricity and ruthlessness. In order to acquire skills and all knowledge necessary for the dominant technology, learning must be mastered and a respectful estimation of masters and teachers is mandatory An appropriate appraisal of incapacities leads to genuine humility, a prerequisite for teachability, but also the basis for genuine appreciation of the skills and creativity of others.

It is easy to imagine that young Isak Borg found in study and all intellectual pursuits a rewarding and satisfying challenge. The isolation of book learning may have offered him a refuge from his siblings and more extroverted peers. With language as a tool, he could give form to his imaginative life with words and take pleasure in the expression of the poets he seems to have enjoyed. Later young Sara says of him, "Isak is enormously refined and moral . . . he wants us to read poetry together . . . he's extremely intellectual." His concentration and hard work in school must have given him considerable prestige at home, as well as advancing his hope of becoming a student of higher learning in the upper levels of academe. It also permitted him to remain the scientifically skeptical, detached observer of others.

At seventy-six, Dr. Borg is physically competent and practical. To have undertaken a fourteen-hour drive, without an apparent moment of doubt in his capacity to manage it alone, offers evidence of his sense of confidence in his physical and mental stamina. He wears glasses only to read and write, smokes little—and then only cigars, "a manly vice." He always has a rope in the back of his car, he claims, in case of need and skillfully manages its deployment after the accident. His skills are not limited to those of the intellect. He even mentions that he takes pleasure now and then in a game of golf.

There can be little doubt as to Dr. Borg's sense of competence in his old age—after all, he is being awarded an honorary doctorate for fifty years of medical practice with distinction. He describes himself as someone wishing to devote himself to "keeping up with the steady progress" made in his profession. "My life has been filled with work and for that I am grateful," he says. In fact, he has taken great pride in his sense of competence, which makes the blow of his failure at his examination by Alman and the verdict of "incompetent" all the more severe.

In reflecting on his whole life, however, one must note that this work competence has been bought and maintained at a high cost. He has undeniably been incompetent as husband, father, and father-in-law. He especially fails Marianne when she comes to him for help. "Don't try to drag me into your marital problems, because I don't give a damn about them —everyone has his own troubles" was his uncaring and prejudiced response. Such an attitude suggests a possibly maladaptive sense of overriding self-satisfaction that tends toward emotional impassivity and dullness.

Adolescence

With emerging adulthood, a young man is challenged to relate to society and its technology and to the world of ideas, ideals, creeds, and symbols. It is important for him to identify himself with life goals worthy of commitment and fidelity and to do this with an appropriate knowledge of his capacities. The sturdy strengths of hope, will, purpose, and competence, which result from the earlier balancing of these stage-specific syntonic and dystonic tensions, will now support these new vital commitments. But this is a demanding step to be taken, and it is easy to become confused and uncertain about one's life role and one's firm sense of "I." There will inevitably arise challenges of loyalty, self-trust in relation to peers, groups, country, and ideals with, one would hope, appropriate mistrust of simplistic approaches and resolutions. Identity confusion with a constant shifting of temporary identities is maladaptive. However, a premature and inflexible commitment may foreclose possible choices of great promise. A total dedication to one cause that is maladaptive for others and oneself may lead to a rigid fanaticism.

Where competencies have been developed and, with them,

predilections that accord with one's capacities and society's needs have been carefully weighed, one's psychosocial identity may initially be wisely molded.

It seems that young Isak Borg made such a felicitous commitment. He had the intellectual capacities for the prolonged and arduous study demanded of the medical profession. He was healthy and strong. He had keen senses and the trained ability to observe with detachment, which, we suspect, he had practiced for many years. He valued scientific inquiry and chose a role of great prestige in the eyes of society and his intellectual peers.

After fifty years of medical practice, he appears to be well satisfied with his choice and his performance; and, indeed, society is ready to bestow on him a high honor in recognition of his professional fidelity.

As he awakens from the first challenging dream sequence early in the morning, he sits up in bed and says, "My name is Isak Borg. I am seventy-six years old. I really feel quite well." On muttering these words, he feels "much calmer." This is surely a statement tantamount to a "station identification." He later tells us that he is the only survivor of ten children, a Lutheran and a Swede, and, above all, a doctor. "If for some reason I would have to evaluate myself," he says, "I am sure that I would do so without shame or concern for my reputation." His sense of his own integrity, at any rate, seems to be high.

However, every man has more than one role to play in life. His work is his professional role. Dr. Borg seems to have sidestepped a real involvement with his many other more personal roles. In an egoistic and single-minded way, he shows no mitigating identity confusion and has experienced little identification with his roles as husband, father, and father-in-law.

In the very first dream, his recognition of the corpse as being himself is obviously startling and painful. He has, old as he is, not yet faced many of the aspects of his personal identity or of his mortality. Indeed, on this very day, when his professional role is supremely confirmed, his own inner sense of identity cohesion, as challenged by his daughter-in-law's confrontation, forces this man to face a certain inner confusion. At this final stage of his life, such confusion could make his generational role highly problematic. But the end of the film indicates some promise of possible new identity potentials in the roles of grandfather and godfather.

Young Adulthood

In reviewing Dr. Borg's life stages, we have indicated how his matrix of personal relationships widened with each step. The circle of potential intimacies has consistently increased to involve caretakers, siblings, extended family, peers, teachers, and the idealized identity models of legend and all literature and history. With adulthood, the individual is first ready for an experience that involves commitment and fidelity capable of culminating in mature love. This presupposes the sharing of life, work, and productivity nurtured by the bond of adult sexuality and a sense of common goals. It therefore demands two already defined identities, neither of which becomes really submerged under the dominance of the other, although each may be both modified and expanded.

We have little evidence in our sparse data of any of Isak Borg's intimate relationships with siblings or friends. Only Sara seems to evoke a deep yearning for a young, caring, feminine figure in his life. This is such a needy, hungry reaching out that it evokes the sound of a crying baby, which is repeated in the film at critical moments of despair. Only with the modern Sara, in his old age, is he able to have a playful relationship, which she induces by her own carefree, humorous manner and spirit.

Indeed, the dystonic elements of isolation and even of exclusivity seem at the sixth stage to be conspicuously prominent. Some exclusivity in intimate relationships, we have postulated, is expectable and sympathic. But too much with little or no intimacy to balance can support a malignant tendency to extreme exclusivity.

Early in the film he says, "I have of my own free will withdrawn almost completely from society." A sweeping relegation of all nonprofessional relationships to the far edges of his life involvements. In his house, he carries on what appears to be a consistently ambivalent relationship with Agda, his faithful housekeeper for some forty years. She maintains order in his environs, freeing his time for walking, golf, and his ongoing professional studies. Is she, perhaps, a replacement for the efficient, bossy, matriarchal aunt of the summer-cottage scenes?

He attempts firmly to keep Marianne at a distance with his unwillingness to listen to her plea for help on her arrival. On the trip, he undertakes to maintain this chill with his cool "Please don't smoke." "There should be a law against women smoking."

His marriage, as he says, was quite unhappy, which is an understatement of the first order, since it was a fiasco and apparently, as his mother suggests, a family disgrace. In this connection, it is interesting to note that during that part of the trip when the Almans live out verbally their miserable relationship for all the occupants of the car to witness, Dr. Borg remains stiffly, dumbly frozen. It is Marianne who takes charge.

After this scene, as he sleeps and dreams of the examina-

tion room where he is failing humiliatingly to answer questions correctly, he demands consideration because he is an
old man with a weak heart. Alman merely answers him,
"There is nothing concerning your heart in my papers."
Indeed, one might say the same of the data concerning his
intimate relationships revealed in this film and its story of his
past. And Alman strikes home cruelly when he adds to his
indictment that Dr. Borg is incompetent because he diagnoses a live woman as dead.

The young Sara tells us how clearly she responds to his
need for her and is also restrained by her respect for his
youthful control and integrity. But she is reaching out for
intimacy and tenderness herself, and he is unable to respond.
Sara says, "Isak is so refined. He is so enormously refined and
moral and sensitive and he wants us to read poetry together
and he talks about the after-life and wants to play duets on
the piano and he likes to kiss only in the dark and he talks
about sinfulness." However, she continues, "But sometimes
I get the feeling that I'm much older than Isak, do you know
what I mean? And then I think he's a child even if we are
the same age. . . ." And again we sense the hunger of young
Isak for the replacement of a very early unrequited love
relationship, about which he remains nostalgic. So Sara is
courted and won by Sigfrid, almost, as she implies, against
her better judgment.

And what may we infer about his choice of a wife? She is
portrayed as a very beautiful and sensuous woman. He still
has her photograph in front of him on his desk. Did he
believe that with such a woman he might overcome the sense
of coldness developing in him as part of his birthright?
Evald's account of himself as "an unwelcome child" with
"indifference, fear, infidelity and guilt feelings" as his
"nurses" does not portray his mother as a warm and mother-

ing person. Needy, passionate, she may have been completely frustrated by the Borg aloofness.

Dr. Borg, the scientist, though obviously drawn to her initially, maintains a professional detachment toward Karin, his wife. She tells us, "Now I will go home and tell this to Isak and I know exactly what he'll say: Poor little girl, how I pity you. As if he were God himself. And then I'll cry and say: Do you really feel pity for me? and he'll say: I feel infinitely sorry for you, and then I'll cry some more and ask him if he can forgive me. And then he'll say: You shouldn't ask forgiveness from me. I have nothing to forgive." How ingrained these words must have been in his memory, since he repeats them verbatim in his dream! Karin is infuriated by the patronizing superiority of these statements and adds, "But he doesn't mean a word of it, because he's completely cold." The husband then becomes doctor and offers to bring her, his patient, a sedative and says he understands everything.

The penalty for such indifferent presumption, Alman says, is "loneliness." Borg is not unmoved and asks, "Is there no grace?" Alman knows nothing about such things and leaves. Isak continues, "I wanted to cry with wild, childish sorrow."

All this is very bleak. However, early in the picture, in the dream sequence about the summer when he observes that he is not present in the birthday scene, he hears someone say, "Isak is out fishing with father," and he says, "Oh, yes, Father and I were out fishing together. I felt a secret and completely inexplicable happiness at this message." Here, then, must have been at least one cherished intimacy of his childhood. If his father, as may be suspected, was also somewhat of an isolate, perhaps this formed a meaningful bond between them.

His acceptance and tolerance of the three young people as they suddenly appear is surprising and heartening. The dreams, the exchange of words with Marianne, and the dreamy fantasy at the summerhouse have already introduced an active leaven.

At the end of the long day, there is considerable evidence that some of his defensive barriers are crumbling. His self-chosen isolation has at least been successfully invaded. But the absence of true intimacy in any relationship has remained his greatest personal defect. In this, he is stagnant, and such a central lack can only impoverish his generational role in adulthood and in old age.

A greater capacity for empathy and playfulness than one might have guessed is reevoked through his sensuous relationship with the three Saras. The reexperiencing through memory and fantasy are apparently strong antidotes for the encroaching despair and possible acceptance of cool numbness in aging that old Mrs. Borg exemplifies.

Adulthood

Now we have reached the years of the stage of generativity, which encompasses a long period of responsibilities demanding stamina and dedication. The challenge is to be productive in all manner of ways, and the strength to be developed is that of care.

Caring embraces taking care of whatever one produces—children, of course, but also all that one does or makes or is part of. It involves playing an active role in the social institutions that create the coherence of a given social structure at a given historical time. Not to be in any way productive and participant in the social network in which one lives and works and loves must result in stagnation—a sense of the end of growth, both personally and as a member of the community and the greater polis.

Whenever and under whatever conditions, the adults of a

given society owe the younger generation the safeguarding of the opportunities and the conditions in which the basic strengths can be developed. They provide the foundations for all future generativity, creativity, and productivity.

We have assumed that young Isak Borg pursued with dedication his own medical training quite early and that he became an excellent family doctor. The testimony of the gas station attendant and his pregnant wife is clear and spontaneous: "Here you see Dr. Borg in person." "This is the man that Ma and Pa and the whole district talk about." "The world's best doctor." And he expresses his nostalgia for those younger days. He looks out at the valley thoughtfully and says, "Maybe I made a mistake." "Perhaps I should have remained here." What a boon in old age to have some element of past generativity acclaimed and applauded. Resting on one's laurels is not altogether supportive unless they are occasionally freshened up.

Dr. Borg is noticeably moved by this encounter, and perhaps pleased that these appreciative remarks have been overheard by his passengers in the car. His young ex-patients, however, draw him back to the present, insisting on making a gift of the tankful of gas and calling attention to the young wife's pregnancy. They even point forward enthusiastically to that future in which their newborn son will be named Isak and he will be asked to stand as godfather for their child.

It is the gas station attendant who assumes that Dr. Borg is about to visit his old mother. Had he really planned to? Certainly, it was not included in the original plan to fly to Lund. But now he and Marianne face this old, isolated woman. Procreative she had been, although perhaps not by choice. Now she is alone and cold. Had she rejected her progeny and the world around her, walled in behind her high enclosure? Or were her aloofness and apparent uncaring so blatant that those who might have played a caring role were repulsed? Marianne, who represents life and vitality, is horrified. Seeing his mother through Marianne's candid eyes and the symbol of the faceless clock shock Isak Borg, whose threshold of vulnerability has already been lowered. They leave arm in arm: she, seeing, perhaps more readily, the source of some of his coolness; he, coping with a glimpse of what his future on his present course could hold. They remain in touch, for later in the story he says to Marianne, "How can I help you?" and even offers, "Won't you have a cigarette?"

But the dystonic has taken its toll—the interest of this only surviving child in his mother has been anything but warm even though he is a physician. His son is more than half frozen and full of hate, and his daughter-in-law is only slowly managing to reengage her father-in-law in vital human relationships. In his many nieces and nephews, he has no interest whatsoever. He says, "I have very little contact with my relatives," and he is the "elder" of a large clan. There are no friends, and he chooses a sterile solitude. This stage of generativity involves the responsibility to care for and care about children, family, work, and community—as the Hindus say, "the maintenance of the world." Since his days of family practice, after which he seems to have become more academic and scientifically oriented, our aging doctor has concentrated exclusively on the maintenance of Isak Borg.

There is, however, a compelling symbol of hope, for Dr. Borg maintains in his household and in his presence a fecund Great Dane bitch obviously the mother of newly dropped puppies—surely an archetypal figure of an undeniably potent canine mother goddess. Did he breed Great Danes and not even mention it as an interest, a very lively involvement for his old age?

Old Age

We have elected *wisdom* as the word that symbolizes the strength of this last stage of the life cycle and have used the words *integrity* and *despair* to represent the opposing poles that characterize the tension in the psyche. *Integrity* we chose because it seems to describe the aging individual's struggles to integrate the strength and purpose necessary to maintain wholeness despite disintegrating physical capacities. It also suggests the need to gather the experiences of a long and eventful life into a meaningful pattern. Old age is a time for remembering and weaving together many disparate elements and for integrating these incongruities into a comprehensible whole. This integrating has been going on throughout the life cycle, especially as each crisis is faced and as strength is generated by the process of resolution itself.

In the same way, elements of despair have inevitably been ingredients of every struggle for balance between the syntonic and dystonic pulls of each stage. To have experienced this world and our human inadequacy to deal with one another and our mutual problems in living and growing is consistently to know defeat. To balance this pull of despair, which may well increase with waning strength, we need to muster all the ingredients of the wisdom we have been garnering throughout the life stages.

Some of these components may be isolated and defined, but the genuinely wise have in some way managed to integrate them all. The oldest and wisest elders understand that situations are complex and that many factors have to be weighed and distinguished. Prejudice is maladaptive and presumptuous, for with age one is forced to concede how little one knows.

This knowledge is the fertile ground (humus) in which

humility and humor are bedded and nourished. Both are vital for survival if the syntonic and dystonic elements are to be balanced and wisdom is to emerge. Resilience to inevitable change and loss is also demanded as a high priority, since this period of life is one of constant adaptation to new situations.

A major challenge is the maintaining of the acuity of the senses so that the body remains actively and safely involved in the affairs of the immediate environment and the larger world and so that relationships remain sensitive, sensual, and sustaining.

How does Dr. Borg measure up to these demanding qualifications of the strength of wisdom? Judged by his own statements, he could be described as both disdainful and presumptuous. To Marianne he says, "I have no respect for suffering of the soul, so don't come to me and complain. But if you need spiritual masturbation, I can make an appointment for you with some good quack, or perhaps with a minister, it's so popular these days." With this statement he mocks Marianne's suffering and annihilates psychiatry as well as the ministry in devastating terms. All this is said before she has really been heard, so that he is guilty of the most careless prejudgment. His disdain for psychiatry and the ministry, two major fields of human care, causes one to wonder about such blatant defensiveness. We learn later what memories he is trying vigorously to wall off from his consciousness.

His embattled yet dependent relationship with Miss Agda points to her as another butt of his scorn. He speaks of her, somewhat his junior, as "that old woman," "that bossy woman," and as an "immensely power-hungry old sourpuss," even when he is talking to himself in his journal.

He knows, it seems at times, little of humility, and yet in his own dream he is deeply humiliated by Alman. It is with the young people that a certain lively humorousness comes into his expression and into his whole benign attitude toward their exaggerated affects and stances.

However, Dr. Isak Borg is still a man of vitality and capable of active involvement in his life and affairs, so there are a number of hopeful signs that he may yet reconcile his life experience and develop a more integral wisdom.

He ruminates at the final ceremony and makes, as he says, "a plan to recollect and write down everything that had happened." "I was beginning to see a remarkable causality in this chain of unexpected, entangled events." Isak Borg has been stimulated into looking at himself and his long life. He prides himself on his ability to probe, to identify, to make a diagnosis. All of the events of the day now being recorded in his journal in such unflattering detail should come to his aid and lead him to new insights.

And the future offers new experiences for self-healing, growth, and change—the more open relationships with his son, with Marianne, even with Agda. And a new generation, a grandson and a godson, will awaken and release perhaps old sources of care, love, and fidelity.

After all, Dr. Isak Borg "feels quite well," as he himself says, and he is only seventy-six years old and a surprisingly resilient man.

The prognosis is encouraging.

Conclusion

"No less than a whole life," we said when choosing to present Bergman's movie. But to this we must eventually add "and not less than a whole communal setting." For it is necessary to permit involvements to assume what we have called the actualized and mutualized character, which alone can make them truly vital. Only in a communal context can we judge how the same individual's relationships have remained developmentally underinvolved or whether, in the course of a lifetime, they have become defensively disinvolved. Furthermore, we have learned that old age brings with it an effort to get reinvolved in typical patterns of living, as it were, in the past.

We have seen how Bergman's moving film confronted Dr. Borg—and us—scene for scene, with the stage-bound involvements of human beings of different ages. This, in fact, has guided us in enumerating those relationships that are ready to evolve from the first to the last stage of development and yet remain apt, in the course of any life history, to become disinvolved—and this to the disadvantage of the individual as well as a loss to all those involved with him. *Disadvantage* can here be too mild a word: we have, in fact, learned to "diagnose" such alienation either as maladaptive, if readaptation is still possible, or as malignant, if something has really atrophied in the person and in his relationships. For, as we must now add, all these stagewise relationships can be truly judged only within the context of the customs of the communal culture; and, indeed, the movie's sequence of scenes tells us a lot about some of the special meanings of the stages as lived in the Sweden of that day. At the end, in the splendid ritual of the Jubilee, and not without our doctor's amused embarrassment, we witness that grandiose ritual display which simultaneously involved not only Sweden's academe but also her nationwide church and even her army's cannons in the honor done to a few truly old medical survivors. Finally, we come to realize that this drama involves us so deeply because the interplay of the grand ritual of a communal ceremony combines with that long day's intimate generational interplay so "naturally" that it draws the old doctor beyond his psychosocial identity into an acute involvement in the problems of his existential identity. However, we will remember that this comes about only because of the determined and vital involvement of his daughter-in-law in her own life crisis of generativity.

IV

Old Age
in Our Society

Every conceptualization of life, so we have claimed, is set forth by some all-inclusive imagery or configuration: ours is the life cycle. In trying to clarify its circular nature, we find the individual life cycle also to be an essential component of the process of innumerable generational cycles. And while this whole process, in its overall rhythm, must follow the reproductive program of organic life, it must, at the same time, persistently work to reconstitute the social order of institutions, in which we must live.

In conclusion, we must go beyond anything the specific data, gathered in as small a group of elders and in as unique a social setting as that of our study, could prove or disprove. In fact, we must appeal to our as yet merely adult readers or perhaps our youthful readers—at any rate, those not yet old readers—to think with us about that expectable old age which is already being formed in today's young people and adults, shaped as we all are by the social conditions and historical relativities of our time.

From the past, from myth and legend, from anthropologists and historians, we learn that the elders of society were the transmitters of tradition, the guardians of ancestral values, and the providers of continuity. They were awarded such titles as sage, patriarch, seer, and venerable counselor and were consulted as advisers and sometimes as prophets, since long-range memories make prediction, founded on experience, trustworthy. Their life histories provided the warp on which the lively threads of the ongoing community were in the process of being woven. This interconnectedness of the social fabric, which stressed the interdependence of all age groups, tended to establish a harmonious wholeness. The philosopher Josiah Royce, writing in the 1880s, tells us, "Therefore the sense of community, the power to work together, with clear insight into our reasons for so working, is the *first* need of humanity." Perhaps what we need today is this "clear insight" into how the elders in our present society can become more integral coworkers in community life. Royce also says that throughout history "all that each age could do was to fund its wisdom into its institutions, its thought, and its art." We question whether this "funding" of the wisdom that perspective provides is sought or welcomed by community institutions, by centers of learning, or in the world of art today.

With the advent of technology and the impact of the values it represents, not only do elders no longer provide continuity, but they also find themselves out of step with their social milieu. Without the technical knowledge and scientific training of their own children and grandchildren, the experiential knowledge they could convey often seems outdated and even quaint. Feeling retired by society, unneeded, and unproductive, they cast about for some comfortable way to "spend" whatever money and time they have in the twenty or more possible years of aging. Maintaining this large "functionless" segment of the population can be a catastrophe for any society.

This predicament is bound to become an increasingly ominous cause for public concern as the statisticians warn us that by the year 2000 at least 30 percent of the population will be over sixty-five years of age. If the prevailing conditions are not rectified, the present working men and women of the world will be looking forward to an initial retirement holiday followed by a dangling and unproductive aging of many years' duration. As elders, they will be forced to watch their own children struggle to maintain a fragmented society and to carry the burden of caring for and educating their children, while bearing the immense expense of supporting a growing population of the aging. For some of these children it will be backbreaking and for others intolerable because of the guilty resentment that will inevitably be aroused.

What can the adults of today do to safeguard their own future and that of their children and grandchildren? Those now fifty years old and facing retirement at sixty-five, in the year 2000, need to begin to meet this very urgent challenge squarely. Old age must be consciously anticipated, and that is why we have to understand the trajectory of the life cycle. Scientists have made great strides in finding cures for many of the diseases that have plagued mankind. Now many more are turning their attention to the prevention and cure of ailments associated with but not intrinsic to aging. As a result of this new concentration of geriatric research, the life span will for many be extended well beyond what was previously expected or planned for the average individual.

The quality of the healthy years added by the extended life span can be drastically improved for all elders. However, such improvement must be planned for if those now in their late forties and early fifties hope to be vitally involved in their later years. What steps can be taken now to ensure that the elderly of the future will remain an integral part of the social fabric?

Retirement

It is generally conceded that, for many professions and many lines of work, retirement is required too early. Naturally, this varies with the individual, but a general rule never covers the needs of a situation that involves so many variables. Some leeway must be possible, for otherwise we tend to accept the lowest common denominator, and that is unjust and unrewarding. As time goes on and the number of older citizens increases and as they become healthier and stronger, these very changes will force a reexamination of the rules now pertaining to retirement. The designation of some age as the norm for this crossing over into old age may be necessary and reasonable. However, one may question the policy that dictates that, regardless of competence and health, the individual may not earn more than a very limited sum without losing his well-earned retirement benefits; it seems both unfair and inimical to all personal enterprise. One may also question the taxation of pension payments that are the reward for years of steady working. Would it not be feasible to allow workers to continue to provide their services? "Networks" of retired ("emeriti") workers have been successfully organized in a number of communities and are a welcome addition to the work force. Sometimes these services involve barter, which is a friendly method of meeting needs all around.

These may all be patchwork suggestions, but we will be obliged to find some specific ways out of a general situation that seems to doom a large segment of our population to inertia and inactivation.

In general, it is true that we do not actually know how competent and industrious people between seventy and eighty years old can be in our society. In an agricultural economy, when they are healthy, they are able to bear a considerable portion of the necessary workload. Old men and women have continued to perform their customary chores until they were physically unable to do so. They sometimes did so of necessity, but more often they seem to have done so by choice. They not only felt useful and needed but actually were. Indeed, if they could express in words what their bodies express in action they would be in agreement with Oliver Wendell Holmes, who in a radio address on his ninetieth birthday (March 8, 1931) said, "The race is over, but the work never is done while the power to work remains. . . . It cannot be, while you still live. For to live is to function. That is all there is in living."

Our technological economy has, as yet, no place for these elders. There is a rumor abroad that in old age one can no longer learn new skills, new approaches to problems, although this has been disproven repeatedly.* It is true that a lifetime of repetitive, dull work will tend to dull one's wits and decrease the motivation to learn—to be curious and inquiring. But exercising the mind refreshes and restimulates it, and in times of need and crisis older people are clearly capable and respond with enthusiasm and energy. You may recall the story of the grandmother cited earlier who took over the care of an infant grandson at her son's request. She reported, "I was his mom. He called me 'Mom.' I took him

---

*See the report of Marian Diamond showing that the brain in old age in an enriched environment is capable of surprising growth. "The Aging Brain: Some Enlightening and Optimistic Results," *American Scientist* 66 (1978): 66–71.

to nursery school with a bunch of kids. I PTA-ed all over again—in my late sixties, this was." This is, of course, an instance of extreme flexibility. Our study gives other examples of elders who pitched in very effectively to care for grandchildren and even ailing relatives.

By relegating this growing segment of the population to the onlooker bleachers of our society, we have classified them as unproductive, inadequate, and inferior. Offering them, on occasions, status honors and honorary memberships shows respect and may be gratifying to them. Taking care of them in innumerable organized ways is being responsible. Entertaining them with bingo games and concerts is, however, patronizing. Surely, the search for some way of including what they can still contribute to the social order in a way befitting their capacities is appropriate and in order.

This leads us back to the mandate of a fixed age for retirement as we now examine its impact on the work force. In the really early years of "old age," beginning after sixty, when retirement is imminent, the aware and thoughtful individual may well begin to realize that a bridge is about to be crossed. In early adulthood, a similar crossing was approached as the individual joined the work force. But this later one is faced with quite different expectations and calls for realistic appraisal and planning. Ideally, clearheaded planning would have brought this change into life cycle perspective years earlier. By their very presence, all elders in the community indicate "loud and clear" that the crossing is ahead and perhaps not far off, but the busy majority of younger adults, inundated with commitments, more often than not remain blind to such evidence.

The moment of retirement itself may be a shocking encounter with the transition about to be made. Many organizations, companies, and professions try to ritualize this moment. The celebration can be festive and more or less ritualized, marking years of service, high achievement, and honorific status. On the other hand, it may take the form of only a final check and a farewell to coworkers bent on emphasizing how fine a life of leisure will turn out to be. However, for the unprepared, for those whose creativity and involvement in work has been of major importance and whose identity is largely derived from that work, there can be a bitter and deprived feeling of being expelled and depreciated. One of our most successful, productively active informants said resignedly, "There's nothing you can do about it. It's like getting the measles." The transition could be substantially eased by a rediagnosis—a redefinition of work that takes into consideration the demands and the pressures on older workers in relation to their physical capacities. For many, an appropriate flexibility of scheduling could be considered, one providing continuity and further commitment to an established field of concentration.

Aside from the damage it does to individuals, our discarding of older workers regardless of their capacities is unrealistic in an economy that needs its most highly trained and creative workers for as long as possible. It is an across-the-board simplification of attitude and practice to devalue wit, creativity, and experience by equating these qualities and weighing them against mere speed and the more up-to-date information of the young.

Given mandatory retirement, though, what can the individual do to maintain vital involvement? For those whose work has been routine and boring, the prospect of meeting with former coworkers outside work hours may provide an ongoing sense of affiliation. They hope to enjoy being free of a physically demanding and disciplined routine. Others may find it involving to give long-needed time to the care of their homes and to relationships with friends and families. But all of these activities are apt to pall in the long run. Like the carefree small dog in Maurice Sendak's *Higglety Pigglety Pop,* these elders may begin to say to themselves, "There must be more to life than this." There is indeed more to life than this, and with some planning and some appraisal of one's capacities, life—especially in the early years of aging— can be full of creative activity and even new work identities. As we noted earlier, our informants report a wide range of activities, some inventively derived from turning old skills into productive new directions like remodeling their homes and rental properties. (Of course, all of this presumes the economic means necessary to support a creative old age.) Some who previously had little time for gardening have become energetic cultivators of exotic plants and landscapers for themselves, their families, and the community. Others have focused their business skills on new enterprises like personal financial investing in real estate and other areas.

Many organizations exist to help older people launch new enterprises and market skills. Volunteer work is desperately needed everywhere in the social order, and there are many opportunities to learn almost anything. Old age is the prime time for individuals to do all the things that the demands of their job made impossible earlier. All of this presupposes that they have managed to maintain reasonably good health and that their previous interests and capacities have remained viable and even lively.

The problems of those over eighty-five are of a different order. We have only begun to recognize their seriousness for these elders and for the social order as their numbers continue to increase. It is now the fastest-growing cohort in the country, and the prognosis is that the increase in numbers will greatly exceed our capacity to care for these elders and to incorporate them into the social fabric.

In a country that has prided itself on independence rather than interdependence, on fresh zest and enthusiasm rather than cautious deliberation, and on agility and buoyancy rather than forthright firmness, the predominant value is, of course, youthfulness. This valuation holds for men in the work world and especially in all technological pursuits and for women in all areas of the social order. It is not surprising, then, that ageism poses such a problem for all older people. Young is beautiful. Old is ugly. This attitude stems from a stereotyping deeply ingrained in our culture and in our economy. After all, we throw old things away—they are too difficult to mend. New ones are more desirable and up-to-date, incorporating the latest know-how. Old things are obsolete, valueless, and disposable. Sometimes they may move into the category of antiques, old ivory, or vintage wines, as do the really old elders, those over ninety-five. Preserved like the antique, the ivory, and the wine, all old persons might present a braver picture, but that takes affluence, luck, and discipline.

The cruelest aspect of this cultural attitude is the elders' vulnerability to the stereotype. Some feel themselves to be unattractive, dull, and, quite often, unlovable, and this depressing outlook only aggravates the problem. One response is to avoid looking or acting your own age at all costs. The result is, of course, humiliating failure. Another attitude is to let go, renouncing even rewarding interests and pleasures as unseemly. The acceptance of the stereotype then actualizes the stereotype itself. Perhaps the middle way is the hardest, since it involves accepting who and what you are with active compliance. This process includes a mature appraisal of being just where you are in the life cycle and an appreciation of the great advantages of this position. An injustice is done to people when they are given so negative a vision of what is ahead in their lives and then not shown how they may more optimally and optimistically plot their course.

The vagueness and insecurity that characterizes old persons who feel it necessary to describe themselves primarily in terms of who they have been is reflected in some of the members of the small sample of elders we interviewed. But, as we have consistently reminded our readers, those in our Berkeley group, though not affluent, were almost all well provided for. Some are perplexed that the end of life has turned out as it has; even where there are complaints, though, there is nonetheless resignation. There is, to our knowledge, no Gray Panther and no member of the Older Women's League (OWL) in the group, no affiliate of the National Council of Senior Citizens (NCSC) or the National Council on Aging (NCOA), and we saw no Senior Power button; the consensus seems to be "Well, that's just how things are." Most of them expressed the feeling of being "lucky."

The majority of elderly people in this country do not enjoy the material security of our Berkeley group. Among the poorest people in any society have always been the elderly, the infirm, and the frail. Even now, in our society, in spite of Social Security benefits, pensions, and Medicare, many elders are among the poorest of the poor—especially the women. In a technological society, all the continuities that offered elders status and even a fringe role as a financially productive worker (farmer, chemist, butcher, baker) have been lost in the vast changes created by a racing technology. The old have thus been forced into the position of supplicants at a point in history when their role identities as storytellers, historians, counselors, and arbiters of disputes have all but disappeared and when their sense of personal dignity is threatened by those who have the power and means to alleviate their needs.

Some efforts have been made to place individuals over sixty years old on the staffs of agencies concerned with aging. The Older Americans Act was amended in 1973 to include a provision for such preferential hiring where agencies were receiving monies under the act. The purpose, the committee report stated, was to "involve senior citizens directly in the development and execution of Title III projects." This would seem to have been a wise and thoughtful decision. However, by 1978 only 6 percent of the staff in the California Department of Aging were over sixty, and some of these elders were only in routine clerical or trainee jobs. There may be valid reasons why this requirement has been disregarded, but the result is that elders are all too regularly treated as clients or even patients in a kindly but deprecating way.

When this becomes the characteristic approach of the caring professions toward the aged, their recourse can only be to pull away, become disinvolved, and more or less accept the stereotype and maintain and entertain themselves as well as their incomes allow. Others give up in less enviable ways, accepting the patient role with bitterness and resignation.

We do, to be sure, have Medicare, which despite its flaws is for old people a lifeline. Medical services of all kinds have so risen in cost that they are beyond the reach of a large segment of the population. This is not the place to debate the virtues of socialized medicine as it exists in European countries, although in many ways it seems to be a more democratic system than our own. In a country that stresses free enterprise, we may well have spearheaded some of the most outstanding innovations in treatment and research. Deplorably, though, this standard of treatment is available only to those who can afford its high costs.

It would be wise and forward-looking for more medical professionals to focus their research on the prevention of those ailments of older people that are not essentially intrinsic to aging itself. Arthritis, heart disease, cataracts, and ear defects, for example, are not necessarily due entirely to the aging process, although the lowered tonus of the body makes it more vulnerable to them. Both arthritis and heart disease may to some degree be checked by appropriate diet. Direct or constant glare, we are warned, induces cataracts, and some ear defects are caused by extremes of intensified sound. Duly informed, we can control some of these factors. Further research will provide more specific guidelines and information. How much more productive and resilient old age could be without some of these ailments, which constrain activities that could otherwise be maintained profitably and creatively for years!

Another important issue is that of the support measures that could keep elders more independently active. Many problems could be taken care of before medical treatment becomes mandatory, but if checkups are not covered by Medicare and if no preventive advice and treatment are available, there remains only the inevitable path to patienthood before belated medical attention is offered.

Many elders, indignant about their enforced powerlessness, join organizations taking on advocacy roles that stress becoming more informed about the world, the nation, the state, and the community in which we live. Such affiliations are supportive both because there is strength in numbers and because they offer the individual active participation in an effort to bring about change in society itself and in the role of elders. This is all to the good and should be encouraged and applauded. It is, however, not reasonable to expect those already old to make drastic changes in either policy itself or in ageism stereotyping in their own lifetimes. The young adults who look ahead, as we have already said, should begin to promote such changes so that social innovations may improve their own lives and those of their children and grandchildren by the time they are elders, in the year 2000.

We have in this century moved from the Thanksgiving-basket brand of philanthropy through the more inclusive social service–Hull House approach, to a national, state, and city awareness of responsibility for the care of the aged. Can we now progress to a genuine valuing of old age, with rights and responsibilities appropriate to the summing up of a lifetime?

Grandparenting

The elders who are the subjects of our study only seldom make explicit their reactions to the stereotyping we have been discussing, and then with little or no emotion. This may at first appear strange, until one remembers that they are not displaced or indigent persons and that most of them take great comfort and pride in their children and grandchildren. After all, they are the century's survivors, who steered their families through three wars and the Great Depression. With only a few exceptions, they feel rewardingly justified and successful in regard to their roles as parents. Most state they have "wonderful" children and even more-remarkable grandchildren. Again, we must point to their fifty odd-year-long relations with the Guidance Study, which encouraged them to focus on parenting and child development. Their conscious, even self-conscious, preoccupation with this aspect of their role identity as "investigated" and "guided" parents is very apparent. This positive appraisal of their success seemed in no way defensive but was, on the contrary, wholeheartedly enthusiastic. Grandchildren and great grandchildren are most often described as perfect.

Photographs of assembled generations suggest great pride in well-played roles as "fledgling ancestors." Since the role of child rearer has been and still seems to be heavily stressed in their lives, it is one element of their identities in which they can take justifiable pleasure. Some statements about these children made by our informants exude a sort of surprised satisfaction: "My sons are all very rich men." "My kids all grew up staunch and sturdy, and have such good characters."

Grandparenting, since it is the culmination of the parenting role, seems to offer elders one of the most positive and vital involvements of old age. Our society, with its tendency to devalue geographical stability and the importance of community, ruthlessly condones the uprooting of families. Bring the young up to be independent, our philosophy seems to say, and you can whisk them anywhere and land them on their feet. Big corporations move their people around on purpose, in order to stress both the dependence of their relationship on the company and their nonattachment to anything that is more important. As a result, the extended family is broken up, and no one has been able to count the cost. Grandparents are often deprived of relationships with grandchildren, whom they scarcely get to know. In an industrial system such as ours, profit making and greed take precedence over other values, such as generational continuity.

Divorce presents another kind of crisis for grandparental relationships. The media have highlighted the pain of those grandparents for whom a child's divorce has meant estrangement from grandchildren. Divorce is, in any case, apt to be a disruptive experience for all concerned. In cases where bitter struggle over the custody of children has ensued and grandparents have taken part in the fray, a retaliatory restriction of visiting privileges has sometimes resulted. In reality, we are told this affects only a small number of people. However, legislation is under consideration to legitimize grandparental claims for contact.

Grandparents have often used this crisis as an opportunity to be helpful by playing an important role in the emotional recovery of children and grandchildren. All too frequently, families in the midst of divorce proceedings become isolated from friends and avoid their previous community supports, such as organizations, churches, and temples. Here the elder generation can play a role, without the usual fear of being intrusive, and help all segments of the family remake their lives. Daughters, and even daughters-in-law, have been helped to return to college or to gain special training so that they can manage independently. (Gone are the days when you simply went back home to your parents under such circumstances.) The provision of child care and of holiday arrangements for children is often welcomed by all concerned. Though older grandparents may feel put upon and too tired to cope with the young, many enjoy this opportunity to give love and support and to play an appreciated and needed role. It is important to note that children of divorce who have been well supported by grandparents have made noticeably better adjustments to living in a broken family situation than have children without grandparental intervention.* Such evidence verifies that the energy and capacity of elders to care for and care about others is available when elders know they are both needed and wanted.

---

*Information provided by Dr. Judith S. Wallerstein, of the Center for Family in Transition. She is the author, with Joan B. Kelly, of *Surviving the Breakup: How Children and Parents Cope with Divorce* (New York: Basic Books, 1980).

Freedom

In old age, serious threats to the autonomy of individuals develop, and they must be recognized as urgent. As we said earlier, all physical disabilities infringe on freedom and self-determination of activity. In a mechanized milieu, the aging individual faces many other limits on the safe range of physical movement. Since many of these restrictions result from sheer thoughtlessness, it may be useful to list a few practical problems that old people confront consistently, and to offer some solutions.

To begin with, adequate protection against violence must be provided and traffic laws strictly enforced so that fragile elders may walk safely in the street. In order to facilitate the use of public buildings (especially registration and polling places) by the elderly, ramps and railings are necessary, as are benches for resting. One of our informants reports very realistically, "I can't even go to the dentist by myself any more. I would walk there, like I always have, but I can't make it without a rest. And there's no place to stop and sit and catch my breath. No benches or seats. Some places don't even have sidewalks. Just more streets than I can walk any more." Clearly, sidewalks in cities, towns, and suburbs should be available to protect all pedestrians, and especially children and elders, from mechanized traffic.

Public transportation must be available for all citizens but, again, especially for those elders who no longer drive. If they are to remain in contact with the activities and involvements that have been and should continue to be a part of their lives, some provisions must be made to render this logistically possible.

The curtailment of older people's participation in the continuing life around them limits their involvement in the give-

and-take of communal life. This curtailment often induces an involuntary withdrawal and is a maladaptation that can all too readily result in inertia and depression.

With aging, as the overall tonus of the body begins to sag and innumerable inner parts call attention to themselves through their malfunction, the aging body is forced into a new sense of invalidness. Some problems may be fairly petty, like the almost inevitable appearance of wrinkles. Others are painful, debilitating, and shaming. Whatever the severity of these ailments, the elder is obliged to turn attention from more interesting aspects of life to the demanding require- ments of the body. This can be frustrating and depressing.

One of our informants states, "As long as you keep in- volved in things, you don't have time to think about yourself or worry about yourself. Now, I've always been too busy to be sitting around. But some of these other people—when groups are hard to get to and activities don't come knocking on their door, why, they just give up. It's kind of sad, really. They're not happy, and there's a lot they could be doing. But they don't seem to fit in anywhere."

With less compassion and more resignation, another infor- mant states, "There is the inclination just to let go . . . to sit here in the evening and watch TV because that is the easiest thing to do. When *you* are over eighty, you'll understand."

Appropriate dependence can be accommodated and ac- cepted by elders when they realistically appraise their own physical capacities. One of our more practical elders simply states, "Of course, you're still interested in everything. But you don't expect yourself to do everything, the way you used to. Some things you just have to let go." However, inappro- priate restriction can be, in its way, insulting and belittling. In describing his current life, one widowed man expresses both his refusal to accept restriction and his willingness to rely on appropriate assistance: "I can stay up here in the woods because I know if I really need help, my son will be here inside of three hours. Now, this deal with fixing my own water pipes, I'd have never tried that without my son so nearby, and I didn't even need him."

Our subjects speak of the importance to them of the independent living they have known and of their real horror of "those homes for the elderly." They feel supported by their familiar settings, by the neighborhood in which they have lived and are known. One woman says somewhat contritely, "I know it would be so much more convenient for them [my family] if I lived nearer, but I'm just not ready to move. I don't want to be a burden out here, and I guess sometimes I am. I just like my independence." Such ruminations, shared by many others, could be paraphrased as follows: "Here I feel independent and in control. Elsewhere I might not make it." It can be ruthless to deprive elders of this sense of secure autonomy in the name of economy and practicality of management. In other parts of the world—in England, Scandinavia, and the Netherlands, for example—home care programs are offered to elders capable of managing at home by themselves, with some help. Meals on Wheels is a step in this direction.

Other policy matters demand attention so that the final years of life may remain as positive and productive as strength permits. One such area of concern is that of housing for the elderly—independent, low-cost housing. Programs are under way but need thoughtful coordination and continuing supervision by a central housing authority. Sensitive questions as to whether elders may or may not be allowed to maintain pets in Housing and Urban Development (HUD) facilities require compassionate as well as practical consideration.

OLD AGE IN OUR SOCIETY

Responsibility

These are all pressing questions for today as well as challenges demanding the attention of those who are currently
involved in the maintenance of our society and who need to
begin to envision their own old age now. It is, on the whole,
easier to recognize problems than to accept responsibilities,
especially when these are not well defined.

As to the elders themselves, what action can they undertake in order to safeguard their independence and sense of
autonomy? Individuals surely owe it to themselves to be as
healthy and as well functioning as possible. However, the
responsibility should not rest entirely with the individuals.
Society owes its citizens encouragement and opportunity to
develop this well-being and should provide as many avenues
as possible for the maintenance of stamina in old age. With
respect to physical well-being, for example, our educational
system could assume much more responsibility for teaching
every child and young person about what their bodies need
for maintenance and long-range survival. Students should be
as diligently trained in good health-maintenance practices as
they are trained in reading, writing, and arithmetic. Anat-
omy and physiology could be curricular subjects of major
interest for all age groups—requiring lifelong learning to
ensure the informed well-being of all members of society.

Currently, our schools do offer physical-education classes
in which exercises are performed. Extracurricular sports are
also available, but here major attention often goes to "the
team," which already excels and is, therefore, the least
needy. Adolescents perhaps have access to a course on "sex"
and on the consequences of intercourse. Childbirth, however,
is not a regular topic of study even though it can be predicted
that one-half of the students will probably bear children. The

result is that young people and even adults can more readily describe mechanical problems in the engines of cars with an adequate vocabulary than find appropriate words for the physical processes of their own bodies. New approaches to the care of the body have in recent years been introduced in educational institutions, in physical-fitness centers, and even in television programs. The benefits to those who have participated prove that such opportunities for learning need to be woven into the larger social system, and perhaps into the time on the job of the working population, as is commonplace in Japan and China.

Given this state of affairs, it isn't surprising that we also receive little instruction about nutrition and the choice and preparation of healthful foods and that our children are the ill-informed victims of television food commercials. The informed intelligence that we need in order to remain unswayed by artfully persuasive mass advertising is not promoted on the lower levels of our educational system.

The fact is we really do not know how well the body can be maintained over the years, or what the potential for the development of physical fitness is or could be. It is clear that dramatic excellence in physical capacity can be the major focus of concentration for only a few individuals. For everyone else, it must go hand in hand with the development of vital mental capacities and work skills.

From infancy on, the senses should be protected and their fullest development encouraged. Are there adequate restrictions against excessive glare and noise, to safeguard the eyes and ears? Do we even know what levels are damaging? Is the light in public buildings, libraries, and schools, in particular, really adequate?

We are learning about pollution of the air we breathe. Is the battle against air pollution as high a priority as it should be? What about smoking in public places and poor ventilation in general?

Our foods are, one might almost say, polluted with sugar and salt and preservatives. Do we exercise enough authority in guarding our food supply, which is now such big business, technologized and politicized? What about tea, coffee, soft drinks, and a number-one killer—alcohol?

We have parks because of the farsightedness of a few heroic ancestors who worked unremittingly to preserve them. As our population increases, however, we will need to protect more of whatever open land still remains unpaved and unpolluted. Parking lots use up the urban spaces where people might be able to move around freely outdoors. City streets do not offer adequate facilities for running, walking, or bicycling, and motorized traffic has the priority at every intersection and crossing.

This indifferent, inattentive society we are belaboring here is, of course, our society—not just U.S., but us. These things need not all be as they are; they can be remedied. In the sixties, there was a voice in the land, a voice for change that protested and offered to lead the way toward better, fuller, richer lives physically and intellectually for us all. Now, facing the longer period of aging in the twenty-first century, we should hear it again.

Those of our elders, our subjects, who worked hard physically through the years and keep it up now more moderately are manifestly sturdy. The couple mentioned earlier who still work on their productive ranch are prime examples of those who have maintained a vibrant health. They are agile and strong and still capable of some hard physical work. The man who has chosen to live in an isolated cabin in the Sierra foothills is also more physically capable and independent than most of his peers. However, others are content to carry on comfortably with a more limited range of activity. Some are devoted to the television set. Their social milieu has not encouraged them to do anything further. They have survived —have done well and are enjoying their years as much as they can. Nothing in their environment stimulates a richer, more abundant life. When they are too frail to care for themselves or are ill, our care facilities will take over. Is that all good enough?

Old bodies can be revitalized through appropriate exercise so that every movement involved in the day's activities can become a pleasure rather than a task. These last years can be more zestful even for those who look to everything else but the use of their bodies to give them a sense of vitality in their lives. It can be done—the body is an ingeniously resil- ient machine. Elders have a responsibility to themselves to maintain their own physical capacities until advanced old age makes them too fragile to exercise the physical autonomy that safeguards independence. Our informants express very clearly their concerns about physical and mental disintegra- tion. "You watch yourself gradually deterioriate, and it makes you mad. Old age is cruel." Nearly all articulate the wish to die before becoming "a real basket case." Another says even more explicitly, "I don't want to linger. No rest home. No convalescent home. I don't want to go on living one minute after I'm mentally or physically incapable."

When individuals can no longer maintain control of their own bodies and need full-time care, the cost is frequently too staggering for the family to bear. The caring institutions of country or state are then the sole recourse. The quality of care offered in such institutions varies enormously. The re- quirements for certification of different categories of care also vary, as do the required qualifications for those in charge of the establishments and of the care. Unfortunately, these homes for the aged are too often run solely as business ventures, and expenditures are minimized for the sake of profit. It is in many ways less costly and more practical to take care of patients on a routine schedule than to allow for individual differences in capacities and needs. The operating of institutions in such mechanical ways degrades both the staff and the patients, since it fails to acknowledge and accommodate the strengths and needs of the individual.

Much thought, effort, and dedication is called for on the part of the caring professions to remedy this regrettable practice, which dehumanizes elderly persons and their caretakers alike.

Lifelong Learning

It is impossible to stress too strongly how important it is that the educational system—schools, junior colleges, universities, and vocational training schools of all kinds—make lifelong learning available to everyone. It is available to all only if it is affordable and if transportation facilities and flexible time schedules exist. The incomes of elders do not permit enrollment in classes with extra charges covering the cost of instruction and of space. Ideally, all higher education courses should be open to elders who bring enthusiasm and interesting perspectives into the classroom. Colleges do offer "emeritus classes" on a number of campuses, but these are often located at quite some distance from the residential areas and the transportation routes. Extension classes of some kind could surely be organized where groups could meet and be stimulated by the scholarship of qualified teachers. Community colleges and many colleges and universities have made it possible for elders and adults to return to school. Both old and young profit from such a mix of ages. These innovations are all to the good.

Most of us have never been in a one-room school where

a variety of age groups are taught together. They still exist in many parts of the world, but we have long since found it more efficient to teach children in peer groups. The disadvantage of this practice is that we seem to proceed after the school age to "peer group" everything we do. Intergenerational groups seldom meet, except when whole families get together. This makes it difficult for individuals either to anticipate the next stage and its challenges or to look back at an earlier one with keenly felt empathy and understanding. For elders this is a deprivation, although many of them may not recognize it as such. To be constantly in the presence of those as old as oneself can be stultifying.

Old people can derive great pleasure from being with younger men and women and can delight in the spontaneous playfulness of children. However, an awkwardness arising from differences in social styles and attitudes can create artificial barriers. An old English widow characterizes the situation with British understatement: "Don't go to these dreadful old folks' clubs, but find some young people. Put up with their casualness."* It could well be claimed that the habitual peer grouping that is so impoverishing for the elderly is at the root of the ageism that besets society today.

When elders are themselves drawn into classrooms to teach youngsters the skills of the past that are being lost in our technological present, they make a valuable contribution. If this somewhat upsets the curriculum, as it well may, it can nevertheless be sufficiently enriching to justify the necessary adjustments of time and schedule. No one would suggest that this can be done in a casual, improvised way. Elders need the support of training in order to be able to

---

*Ronald Blythe, *The View in Winter: Reflections on Old Age* (New York and London: Harcourt Brace Jovanovich, 1979), 266.

transmit skills effectively, and classroom teachers need to practice the art of cooperating with them. But what needs to be developed in everyone involved is the attitude of mind that acknowledges contributions of elders as a worthy and valued gift.

Arts

In general, the school curriculum focuses on giving future citizens the skills for taking part in the existing social order and on preparing them for work roles in adult life. This is necessary, of course. Given a broader, more encompassing view of the whole life cycle, the arts provide a curriculum that can be enriching throughout every stage of life, offering a broader range of study experience for pupils of varying capacities and potentials. In our schools, the arts tend to be treated as unimportant, adjunctive areas of special interest. In colleges, they become preparatory courses for professional training. Many young people have no art experience in their student years, probably because it does not seem to promise a lucrative work life.

At retirement, with no previous experience in art activities, an individual is likely to find it hard to move into the specialized fields of art. An opening up of this area of creativity and stimulation can greatly enrich the elder both intellectually and aesthetically. In fact, just because these activities have remained outside the average experience of the individual, they offer new territory for investigation and enrichment. They demand an involved immersion in sensory awareness for which the often overcommitted, middle-aged adult could not find time but in which the retiree is free to engage.

Many people think they have no creative ability, but this

is largely the result of cultural conditioning. Almost every-one can experience the creative stimulus of participation in music, dance, painting, and sculpture, not to mention drama, which, like ritual and carnival, can combine all the media—a natural and enriching interweaving that enhances them all. For the aging, participation in these expressions of artistic form can be a welcome source of vital involvement and exhil-aration. Our social order does not make such enrichment easily available. But it can be provided, with a bit of imagina-tion and ingenuity, in many situations when the energies and enterprise of a few enthusiasts support the effort. Take a room, a barn, a warehouse, and hang the walls with finished and unfinished paintings and drawings. Materials of great variety and texture—metal, fiber, clay, wood, and stone—should welcome even those on walkers, on crutches, and in wheelchairs. Of course, guides would be present to show how the fibers can be woven, knitted, knotted into interesting forms; the metals cut, bent, enameled; the wood filed, sanded into a fine sheen; and the clay hand-shaped or molded on a wheel. There would also be music, singing, and body move-ment with rewarding surprises for those no longer feeling in charge of their own bodies. Poetry and writing of all kinds could have their place, and drama enacted or read could offer the players defined roles.

This is a setting in which every sense can be stimulated—sight, hearing, touch, taste, smell, and the kinetic sense of the entire musculature. It should be antithetical, in every way, to what one old man has described as a "thinning of the sense of life by loss of objects and interests."* Nothing could be more conducive to keeping elders in touch with the material world and their whole sensory being. The aging individual

---

*Quoted in Blythe, *The View in Winter,* 242.

needs the satisfaction of feeling that these sensory antennae, on which we all rely throughout life, are doing their utmost to alert and empower the aging body to remain an actively involved, as well as creative, agent in the world of people and materials.* In itself this should be a reason not to limit old people to a peer group milieu, since aging is a dead end as a topic and can be lightened and countered only by rather forced humor. "When the involvement is checked and curtailed, energy becomes deflected into channels unaccustomed to receive it, those of the self when brought to a standstill. This unfamiliar and usually unattractive self hypnotises the old man or woman," says an observant old teacher.† One of our informants says decisively, "As long as you keep yourself involved in things, you . . . keep your mind occupied so you don't have time to think about yourself or worry about yourself. Once you give in, you're lost."

Rather than leaving old people uninvolved with nothing to think about except their own deterioration, we should foster the delight and involvement of the senses in such a setting as a lively studio workshop.

In such a milieu of stimulus and response with active involvement, there is little time or occasion for the wearying and sometimes self-pitying rumination about or discussion of ailments. When young people—or any other generation, especially children —are also involved, the change in the mood of elders can be unmistakably vitalizing.

A studio workshop where dedication to the process and the project is the center of attention for those involved is no place for commiseration, for the discussion of symptoms and disabilities. The reason for this is not hard to find. There are

---

*Joan M. Erikson, *Activity, Recovery, Growth: The Communal Role of Planned Activities* (New York: W. W. Norton, 1976).

†Quoted in Blythe, *The View in Winter,* 257–58.

no listeners, and nothing is more discouraging to the complainer than a would-be audience of workers entirely preoccupied with materials, tools, and processes.

We have splendid museums both large and small. Many of the most avid art collectors of the world are among the elders of our society. It may be that elders should not be expected to function as active, fund-raising members of the board, since this can be arduous labor of the sort that may well have been an integral part of their previous adult maintenance of the world. However, a council of elders would offer amateurs (lovers of art) the opportunity to express their views concerning policy and their informed opinion on some of the selection processes of the institution. For the participating elders, such activities provide genuine status and the legitimate sense of being a competent member of a cultural enterprise that values the transmission of culture and continuity through its elders. One of our senior subjects, as we reported earlier, was, until recently, an active docent in a San Francisco museum and derived, and undoubtedly gave, great pleasure from this volunteer work.

There could also be programs in which elders interplay with younger adults and children in studying the exhibits and taking part in art experiences related to the theme of the display. In one museum, this is being programmatically organized with noteworthy success. Through these activities, it is hoped, both young and old will be encouraged to make more profitable use of what the museum has to offer and "elders are given the opportunity to resume the role of elders and teachers."*

This pilot project, now in its second year, has drawn many

---

*Interview with Helaine Fortgang, director, Jewish Community Museum, San Francisco.

old and young into the museum and has been enthusiastically supported by the museum staff as well as by grants from the California Arts Council and the National Endowment for the Arts. Is this not an important intergenerational contribution that other museums might realistically emulate?

As was mentioned earlier, for elders to be included as contributing participators in the life of museums large and small, appropriate consideration for their physical needs must be given and the cost to them kept minimal.

The same is true of theater, where all of life's stages are played by characters who act out their stresses, their conflicts, and even, perhaps, their accruing strengths. Many elders who have lived through so much of the life cycle express a particular sensitivity or appreciation for dramatic characterization. Human foibles, self-deceptions, and pretenses are far more accessible to the discerning eye that casts a long backward glance and responds empathically. But, once again, low-priced admission and easy transportation must be arranged.

Drama groups for elders, too, offer involvement that could be especially enlivening. They have been successfully organized and give promise of synthesizing for many older people a good number of the forms and media of art experience. In fact, an upsurge of interest in the organization of senior dramatic groups has occurred in the last decade. The American Theater Association publishes the *Senior Adult Theater Information Network,* which includes a fascinating listing of the names of senior groups, including Tale Spinners, Spice, Improvise, Autumn Players, and Senior Stars. At present, twenty senior drama programs and many other workshop groups and short-term projects are noted. SAT (Senior Adult Theater) promotes an intergenerational approach that has proven to be highly rewarding. The acting out of earlier life stages in creative drama should be a meaningful art experience for elders, in coming to terms with the human life cycle.

Much evidence is available demonstrating that the graphic arts are areas of genuine involvement and accomplishment for elders. Outstanding American senior artists like Georgia O'Keeffe, Robert Motherwell, Dick Kunig, and Alice Neel immediately come to mind. Ever since Grandma Moses startled the world with her artistry and expertise, those who have worked with elders and painting have expressed amazement at how quickly they can free themselves to respond to the medium with integrity and a unique personal style. From Paris, we have the report and publication of a major exhibit devoted to the art of elders, demonstrating their capacity to create artwork of "a different class altogether from the achievements of casual or amateur artists." Workshops in painting and sculpture were established by Dr. R. Laforestrie at the Charles Foix Hospital in Ivry, followed by an exhibit of the work of these elders.* Three members of the staff report, "The experiences with painting and sculpture which have been a true adventure for all of those involved, forces us to re-evaluate the aging process and to get rid of all preconceptions, stereotyped ideas and caricatures which tend to warp our dynamic and positive view of life."†

After this exhibit came several others, sponsored by smaller galleries in Paris. This kind of supportive display of fine work could do more than many words to encourage older people to develop latent capacities and to be enriched in the process.

The verbal arts, too, are the province of the elderly, who

---

*A catalog illustrated in color recorded this event, and a paper offered by R. Laforestrie, A. Lizotte, and R. Moulais to the Thirteenth International Congress of Gerontology describes the work.

†Bernard Colin, Renne La Forestrie, and Prof. Robert Moulias, chief of geriatric service, Charles Foix de Ivry Hospital.

have stories of a world and a life that have all but disappeared. They should have opportunities to tell these tales because they enrich us all and because, in the telling, the elders remember and recollect their lives. Such memories are often more vivid than recent events, perhaps because their senses were then so vitally involved and have kept those sensory images vibrant. A long life cycle can be reviewed more effectively in this way than when it is remembered piecemeal and by chance.

Those who have worked with elders in freeing them to write narrative or poetic reminiscences of their lives have been amazed at their capacity to express themselves. As one might guess, the result is a heightened sense of aliveness and vitality in these elders, many of whom have been in nursing homes or in care facilities—for a number of years.*

Artists in Old Age

Simone de Beauvoir, in her monumental work on old age, has assembled numerous statements by old artists—writers and painters who record their sense of newfound creativity and impetus in the later years of their lives. Whitman's testimony is particularly moving since he was in very poor physical health and finally was confined to a wheelchair. His mind, however, was clear, and he still had the use of his right arm. "Now that I am reduced to these two things, what great wealth they are!" he wrote. ". . . But as life wanes, and all the turbulent passions calm . . . Then for the teeming quietest, happiest days of all!"† A touch of bravado perhaps, but gallant!

---

*Kenneth Koch, *I Never Told Anybody: Teaching Poetry Writing in a Nursing Home* (New York: Random House, 1978).

†From a letter by Whitman, quoted in Simone de Beauvoir, *The Coming of Age*, trans. Patrick O'Brian (New York: Putnam, 1972), 310.

Not all the writers de Beauvoir quotes join these ranks, but the painters who pioneered the renaissance of their art in the early years of this century offer us an amazing record of continuing creativity and effective, consistent industriousness. It has also often been observed how persistently involved in their work and performance many musicians have been. Conducting an orchestra is a strenuous activity, and the practice and performance schedules are rigorous. The motivation of these artists seems phenomenal, and few even broach retirement at the age of sixty-five or seventy-five.

As we see it, and as many of our subjects demonstrate, the early years of the long span of aging are open for creative living: experimentation with new life-styles or exploration of new activities that can become important involvements or perhaps only a delightful expansion of one's range of interest and appreciative experience.

Vital Involvement

From our experience and work in human development and our interviews with elders, we have selected a major theme for our presentation because it has proven especially illuminating and useful in our understanding of old age. As the title of our book indicates, this theme is *involvement,* and we have stressed the meaning of this word and its significance throughout life. That this involvement must be vital and include mutuality of experience is also one of our precepts; this is not surprising, since vitality is the very breath of the life force itself.

How vitally involved are our Berkeley elders in the activities of their old age? The question is difficult to answer. As we have indicated, many of these elders are involved in a diversity of activities and relationships. Others present a very different picture. A few have remained active with some facet of their previous occupations. The women, of course, are still busy with household affairs. With some outside help and some cooperation from their retired husbands, they shop, cook, wash dishes, and "clean up" in general. A few of the men do a little gardening, make repairs in the house, and take part in an interesting pastimes previously enjoyed. One or two men and women attend club meetings or take part in church activities. Several go occasionally to the theater or a concert and make short trips. All watch television. Who can measure whether this preoccupation is "good" or "bad"? (It entertains and passes the time and, at best, keeps the watcher in touch with the wider world, but it does demand much sitting and straining of the eyes.) Certainly, it exists, and for better or worse, television appears to be here to stay.

It seems impossible not to ask ourselves, Is this enough? Here again the issue of the elderly and the community organization arises in regard to the need to reach out to our elders and to include them more effectively. For the most part, these old people are not even housebound. Do they have nothing to offer? Is there nothing the social milieu, the community, can or should ask of them? They have traveled a long and often difficult road. Is their experience of no value to younger people? Socrates said in *The Republic*, "I consider the old who have gone before us along a road which we must all travel in our turn and it is good we should ask them of the nature of that road." Perhaps Socrates did listen and thus formulated his wise, simple, thought-provoking questions for the attending Greek scholars and philosophers. How can we have readier access to such wisdom for our way?

A few of our old people speak of being ready and willing to die. One remarks, "When you get to my age, why, I am willing to die any time. The only thing that keeps me alive is my obligation to the family." Some even would prefer "not to go on." Another states humorlessly, "You have had your life and lived a long time. You know the saying 'The good die young.' Well, I must have been terribly bad in my youth, because I am still living." Most, however, seem to savor their sensory attachment to life even when that life is rather inactive.

The major involvement that uniformly makes life worth living is the thought of and participation in their relationships with children and grandchildren. Their pride in their own achievement in having brought up their young, through thick and thin, and their satisfaction in the way these young have developed gives them, for the most part, deep gratification. With the arrival of grandchildren, they may identify themselves as ancestors, graduated to venerability. Listen to their voices as they trace their own ancestry and that of their children's traits: "She has her mother's fire, that first girl of ours. She has more energy and more projects than anyone. Come to think of it, my mother had that fire, too. And my wife's two grandmothers." "My son is a perfectionist, like me." "The kids are innately smart, like their father."

This enthusiasm for procreativity, as we mentioned earlier, is so outspoken in our group of elders probably because they have participated for nearly sixty years in a study whose main focus was their children. But it is a natural enthusiasm for all parents and perhaps especially for grandparents. Before we were, there were ancestors—when we leave, there will be descendants and/or memorable deeds and accomplishments.

Perhaps in the not-too-distant future, when there are more healthy, vital old people who look forward with anticipation and pleasure to a long life, all of the aspects of purposeful involvement discussed in this section will be taken as a matter of course. In the meantime, we must press on to the point where those now fifty can look forward to a life much richer than that of today's older people, who must invest so much energy in opening doors now closed to them.

The Life Cycle

The life cycle, however, does more than extend itself into the next generation. It curves back on the life of the individual, allowing, as we have indicated, a reexperiencing of earlier stages in a new form. This retracing might be described as a growth toward death, if that did not ring false as a metaphor. Maples and aspens every October bear flamboyant witness to this possibility of a final spurt of growth. Nature unfortunately has not ordained that mortals put on such a fine show.

As aging continues, in fact, human bodies begin to deteriorate and physical and psychosocial capacities diminish in a seeming reversal of the course their development takes. When physical frailty demands assistance, one must accept again an appropriate dependence without the loss of trust and hope. The old, of course, are not endowed with the endearing survival skills of the infant. Old bodies are more difficult to care for, and the task itself is less satisfying to the caretaker than that of caring for infants. Such skills as elders possess have been hard won and are maintained only with determined grace. Only a lifetime of slowly developing trust is adequate to meet this situation, which so naturally elicits despair and disgust at one's own helplessness. Of how many elders could one say, "He surrendered every vestige of his old life with a sort of courteous, half humorous gentleness"?

We do not yet know, and it is important for us to know that we don't know, just what the timing is for the optimal maintenance of human bodies. It remains to be demonstrated what role willpower and the determination to extend the years of vitality may play in such an extension. Here there is much to learn about the potential for increased vitality during the years of aging.

We do know, however, that the adaptation of individuals to the needs of the body, the community, and the environment in which they live is mandatory for survival. Maladaptation at any stage of the life cycle can impair development and devitalize both the individual and, by association, the community. Earlier, we considered both maladaptive and malignant tendencies in the development of the life process. Let us now attempt to identify in greater detail the adaptation, maladaptation, or malignancy of certain tendencies in the final stage of life. This should not be confused with a review or appraisal of values and virtues. Here we are discussing survival skills and not character strengths or deficiencies.

What is adaptation, and what does it demand of human or beast or even vegetable? It demands, first of all, that the animal or plant accept the place where it happens to be. Human beings and, of course, many animals have more volition regarding their habitat, but even that is limited. Acceptance involves adjustment to place and to the natural and man-made forms and forces that are a part of it.

Since all matter is in some way interconnected, it is clear that an interdependence is mandatory even for mere survival. It is fascinating that we, as a people, should cling so tenaciously to our pipe dream of independence as we become increasingly dependent on our interconnectedness. Such a web so binds us that we are fully dependent on these connections for all our basic needs—light, energy, shelter, transportation, and food. Gone are the days of the log cabin, the garden, and the farmyard, when independence seemed feasible. The network of which we are a part is not local but nationwide and, indeed, now worldwide. Can we not sense this interdependence and teach our children in such a way that they may value relatedness more highly and see better how closely the people of the world are bound together? Surely, our one hope for the future of humankind is in the recognition and acceptance of this interdependence as our only survival course for the planet. This interdependence in turn demands a kind of resilience on the part of the individual, an evolving of appropriate behaviors. At best, this relatedness will be evolved creatively, even playfully, within the capacities and limitations of that which would adapt. For human beings, this would seem to call for imaginative initiative under the guidance of resilient trust with a realistic ratio of mistrust. Need one say that the senses should be acute and that alertness to constant change demands an awareness of all the interdependent entities of the situation? All of this calls for a supple mind, an openness to potentialities, and a dependence on sturdy physical organisms with the skills to carry out or modify the ideas that are generated. For the elderly, then, adaptation poses a greater challenge, and society and individual communities need to find ways to meet that challenge.

So here we are, nearing the end of the twentieth century, and we have a new and rather alarmingly large number of elders, many of whom may be alive until they are ninety or more years old. This poses new problems for the world and for them. Few guidelines are available, but perhaps the laws of adaptation in the service of survival may open our minds to new strategies.

Earlier we considered some of the malfunctioning of the social order in respect to the care for and the rights of senior citizens, the malignant carelessness in the supervision of nursing homes for the elderly, the maladaptive arbitrariness of retirement regulations, and the lack of consideration for the transportation of those who can no longer drive or even walk or climb steps without appropriate safety measures.

But let us turn our attention to the elders themselves and consider what attitudes and behavior are maladaptive for old people in their social settings at this time and in this country. No doubt, every social agency that has dealings with older people would have its own list of uncooperative stances, but for the moment we must generalize.

Possibly the most malignant tendency of elders is what might be called a truly obstinate refusal to accept obvious symptoms of deterioration. Consider the woman described earlier who refuses to use a wheelchair and insists on walking with only a cane. But since she really cannot walk far that way, she rarely moves beyond her bed, bathroom, and breakfast bar. This stubbornness interferes with appropriate medical and therapeutic interventions, even with those available through clinical facilities and nursing care. Such refusal is apparent in a failure to take responsibility for physical needs —nutrition and exercise—and a disdainful lack of appreciation of the danger to oneself and others when the deterioration of the senses should preclude, for example, driving and bicycling.

Less obvious tendencies, though certainly malignant when overdetermined, are surliness and persistent self-pity. In addition, disdain may hold the potential help of others at a distance, and a pompous pretension to wisdom or integrity, merely on the basis of age, may also serve to isolate. A withdrawn, mistrusting despair makes unrewarding labor of the needed assistance offered by caretakers.

To fail to press for ever-renewed integration in the face of disintegration is maladaptive and is apparent in those who accept the stereotype of aging as patienthood. On the other hand, a denial of the decline of stamina and competence inhibits elders from taking the necessary personal responsibility for their own physical well-being and the exercise of their intact capacities. It also prohibits the maturation of mutuality and interdependence in old age.

A realistic despair about the world and so-called progress is only reasonable, but when this reaches a point of inactivating the individual, it can surely be maladaptive. The fear of the dependence that accompanies infirmity, combined with the original and earliest fear of abandonment, is one that can be met only with the accrued trust and faith of a lifetime and with the support of those who care and are responsible.

The infant, we said, *must* develop some trust in order to survive, and its development is a mandatory survival skill. For the mother or caring person, the infant's helplessness is an instinctive claim on her responsive care—the eye-to-eye contact that, evoked very early, forms a lasting bond of mutuality. In the case of "normal" and healthy children, the soft and perfect small body is an aesthetic pleasure to tend. The smile captivates and the fingers that so early grasp and reach out to touch evoke a mutual trust between adult and infant.

Elders have both less and more. Unlike the infant, the elder has a reservoir of strength in the wellsprings of history and storytelling. As collectors of time and preservers of memory, those healthy elders who have survived into a reasonably fit old age have time on their side—time that is to be dispensed wisely and creatively, usually in the form of stories, to those younger ones who will one day follow in their footsteps. Telling these stories, and telling them well, marks a certain capacity for one generation to entrust itself to the next, by passing on a certain shared and collective identity to the survivors of the next generation: the future. Trust, as we have stated earlier, is one of the constant human values or virtues, universally acknowledged as basic for all relationships. Hope is yet another basic foundation for all community living and for survival itself, from infancy to old age. The question of old age, and perhaps of life, is how—with the trust and competency accumulated in old age—one adapts to and makes peace with the inevitable physical disintegration of aging.

After years of collaboration, elders should be able to know and trust, and know when to mistrust, not only their own senses and physical capacities but also their accumulated knowledge of the world around them. It is important to listen to the authoritative and objective voices of professionals with an open mind, but one's own judgment, after all those years of intimate relations with the body and with others, is decisive. The ultimate capacities of the aging person are not yet determined. The future may well bring surprises.

Elders, of course, know well their own strengths. They should keep all of these strengths in use and involved in whatever their environment offers or makes possible. And they should not underestimate the possibility of developing strengths that are still dormant. Taking part in needed and useful work is appropriate both for elders and for their relationship to the community.

With aging, there are inevitably constant losses—losses of those very close, and friends near and far. Those who have been rich in intimacy also have the most to lose. Recollection is one form of adaptation, but the effort skillfully to form new relationships is adaptive and more rewarding. Old age is necessarily a time of relinquishing—of giving up old friends, old roles, earlier work that was once meaningful, and even

possessions that belong to a previous stage of life and are now
an impediment to the resiliency and freedom that seem to be
requisite for adapting to the unknown challenges that determine the final stage of life.

Trust in interdependence. Give and accept help when it is
needed. Old Oedipus well knew that the aged sometimes
need three legs; pride can be an asset but not a cane.

When frailty takes over, dependence is appropriate, and
one has no choice but to trust in the compassion of others
and be consistently surprised at how faithful some caretakers
can be.

Much living, however, can teach us only how little is
known. Accept that essential "not-knowingness" of childhood and with it also that playful curiosity. Growing old can
be an interesting adventure and is certainly full of surprises.

One is reminded here of the image Hindu philosophy uses
to describe the final letting go—that of merely being. The
mother cat picks up in her mouth the kitten, which completely collapses every tension and hangs limp and infinitely
trusting in the maternal benevolence. The kitten responds
instinctively. We human beings require at least a whole lifetime of practice to do this. The religious traditions of the
world reflect these concerns and provide them with sub-
stance and form.

The Potential Role of Elders in Our Society

Our society confronts the challenge of drawing a large
population of healthy elders into the social order in a way
that productively uses their capacities. Our task will be to
envision what influences such a large contingent of elders
will have on our society as healthy old people seek and even
demand more vital involvement. Some attributes of the ac-

crued wisdom of old age are fairly generally acknowledged and respected. If recognized and given scope for expression, they could have an important impact on our social order. We suggest the following possibilities.

Old people are, by nature, conservationists. Long memories and wider perspectives lend urgency to the maintenance of our natural world. Old people, quite understandably, seem to feel more keenly the obstruction of open waterfronts, the cutting of age-old stands of trees, the paving of vast stretches of fertile countryside, and the pollution of once clear streams and lakes. Their longer memories recall the beauty of their surroundings in earlier years. We need those memories and those voices.

With aging, men and women in many ways become less differentiated in their masculine and feminine predilections. This in no way suggests a loss of sexual drive and interest between the sexes. Men, it seems, become more capable of accepting the interdependence that women have more easily practiced. Many elder women today, in their turn, become more vigorously active and involved in those affairs that have been the dominant province of men. Some women come to these new roles by virtue of their propensity to outlive the men who have been their partners. Many younger women have made a similar transition by becoming professional members of the work force. These women seem capable of managing parenting and householding along with their jobs, particularly if they have partners who learn cooperation in these matters as an essential component of the marriage contract.

Our subjects demonstrate a tolerance and capacity for weighing more than one side of a question that is an attribute of the possible wisdom of aging. They should be well suited to serve as arbiters in a great variety of disputes. Much experience should be a precursor of long-range vision and clear judgment.

The aged have had a good deal of experience as societal witnesses to the effects of devastation and aggression. They have lived through wars and seen the disintegration of peace settlements. They know that violence breeds hatred and destroys the interconnectedness of life here on our earth and that now our capacity for destruction is such that violence is no longer a viable solution for human conflict.

Ideally, elders in any given modern society should be those who, having developed a marked degree of tolerance and appreciation for otherness, which includes "foreigners" and "foreign ways," might become advocates of a new international understanding that no longer tolerates the vicious name-calling, deprecation, and distrustfulness typical of international relations.

It is also possible to imagine a large, mature segment of the aging population, freed from the tension of keeping pace with competitors in the workplace, able to pursue vigorously art activities of all varieties. This would bring an extraordinary liveliness and artfulness to ordinary life. Only a limited portion of our adult population now has either the time or the money to be involved in activities of art expression or as appreciative supporters of the performing arts. Widespread participation in the arts is possible only if children are encouraged to develop those roots of imaginative play that arise from stimulating sensory experience. Elders learn this as they undertake to open these new doors of experience and could promote the inclusion of the arts in the educational system. The arts offer a common language, and the learning of that language in childhood could contribute to an interconnection among the world's societies.

The development of a new class of elders requires a continued upgrading of all facilities for the health care and education of people at all stages of life, from infancy to old age. Organisms that are to function for a hundred years need careful early nurturing and training. Education must prepare the individual not only for the tasks of early and middle age but for those of old age as well. Training is mandatory both for productive work and for the understanding and care of the senses and the body as a whole. Participation in activities that can enrich an entire lifetime must be promoted and made readily available. In fact, a more general acceptance of the developmental principle of the life cycle could alert people to plan their entire lives more realistically, especially to provide for the long years of aging.

Having started our "joint reflections" with some investigation of the traditional themes of "ages" and "stages," a closing word should deal with the modern changes in our conception of the length and the role of old age in the total life experience. As we have described, modern statistics predict for our time and the immediate future a much longer life expectancy for the majority of old individuals rather than for a select few. This amounts to such a radical change in our concept of the human life cycle that we question whether we should not review all the earlier stages in the light of this development. Actually, we have already faced the question of whether a universal old age of significantly greater duration suggests the addition to our cycle of a ninth stage of development with its own quality of experience, including, perhaps, some sense or premonition of immortality. A decisive fact, however, has remained unchanged for all the earlier stages, namely, that they are all significantly evoked by biological and evolutionary development necessary for any organism and its psychosocial matrix. This also means that each stage, in turn, must surrender its dominance to the next stage, when its time has come. Thus, the developmental ages for the pre-adult life stages decisively remain the same, although the interrelation of all the stages depends somewhat on the emerging personality and the psychosocial identity of each individual in a given historical setting and time perspective.

Similarly, it must be emphasized that each stage, once given, is woven into the fates of all. Generativity, for example, dramatically precedes the last stage, that of old age, establishing the contrast between the dominant images of generativity and of death: one cares for what one has generated in this existence while simultaneously preexperiencing the end of it all in death.

It is essential to establish in the experience of the stages a psychosocial identity, but no matter how long one's life expectancy is, one must face oneself as one who shares an all-human existential identity, as creatively given form in the world religions. This final "arrangement" must convince us that we are meant as "grandparents," to share the responsibility of the generations for each other. When we finally retire from familial and generational involvement, we must, where and when possible, bond with other old-age groups in different parts of the world, learning to talk and to listen with a growing sense of all-human mutuality.

Index

napping, 190
National Endowment for the
Arts, 321
National Institute of Mental
Health, 20
nature, faith in, 225–26
Neel, Alice, 322
neighbors, caring for, 100
networks, 127
of retired workers, 296
neurosis, 41
nuclear war, 67–68
nurturing, 73, 75, 92, 102–3
nutrition, 312, 313, 330

Oakland Growth Study, 17
Oedipus complex, 241, 275
O'Keeffe, Georgia, 322
old age, elders:
advice offered by, 68–69, 87–88
in agricultural economy, 297
anticipation of, 56, 295
coming into one's own in,
180–81
communal involvement in,
50–51
continuity provided by, 294
cultural prejudices about, 301–2
over eighty-five, 300–301
existential integrity of, 14
as "functionless," 294–95, 298
integration processes in, 70–72
of "Isak Borg," 288–90
models for, 56–60
planning in, 65
planning of, 14, 298, 300
potential role of, 333–37
psychosocial development in,
37–38
in social perspective, 61–62
stereotypes about, 301–2, 303,
305
time sense in, 58

youth compared to, 60
see also specific topics
Older Americans Act, 303
open-mindedness, 60–61
optimism, 63, 67–68
oral stage, 34, 48

painting, 322, 324
parents:
advice offered by, 87–89
guilt of, 81
informants' emphasis on role
as, 75–76
as models for old age, 57–58
surrogate, 94, 297–98
parks, 313
partial-care facilities, 28, 201
patience, 60, 69
peer groups, intergenerational
groups vs., 316, 319
Pennsylvania, University of,
Rehabilitation Research and
Training Center of, 20
personal space, 27–29
philosophy of life, 218
generativity and, 101–4
identity and, 139–40
photographs, 28
identity and, 137
physical deterioration:
accommodation to, 191–94
autonomy and, 189–200, 216–17
competence and, 165–67
denial of, 330
eye problems and, 190, 192–93,
195
freedom and, 309
hearing impairment and, 190,
233, 304
identity and, 130–31
impairment vs. disability or
handicap, 193–94, 198
initiative and, 170, 180